BACTERIOLOGY RESEARCH DEVELOPMENTS

LEPROSY

FROM DIAGNOSIS TO TREATMENT

Bacteriology Research Developments

Additional books in this series can be found on Nova's website under the Series tab.

Rare Disorders Research Progress

Additional books in this series can be found on Nova's website under the Series tab.

BACTERIOLOGY RESEARCH DEVELOPMENTS

LEPROSY

FROM DIAGNOSIS TO TREATMENT

DANIEL L. KNUTH
EDITOR

nova
Medicine & Health
New York

Library of Congress Cataloging-in-Publication Data

ISBN: 978-1-53616-629-3
Library of Congress Control Number:2019953071

Published by Nova Science Publishers, Inc. † New York

CONTENTS

PREFACE

Leprosy: From Diagnosis to Treatment discusses the current public health challenges in leprosy control face, exploring opportunities that may potentially accelerate progress towards the elimination of leprosy.

Leprosy is the least contagious of infectious diseases; it is caused by *M. leprae* and *M. lepromatosis* and mainly affects the skin and peripheral nerves. In addition to existing interest due to the variation in the clinical characteristics of the disease between people, the immune response in this pathology will also differ.

In the course of the disease, leprosy patients can experience episodes of acute inflammatory reactions known as leprosy reactions. Leprosy reactions are complications that may occur before, during, or after treatment, and cause further neurological damages that can cause chronic disabilities. As such, the authors discuss the role of immune response in leprosy pathogenesis and leprosy reactions.

The treatment of leprosy is always based on the final clinical and laboratory confirmation of the diagnosis. The diagnosed patient must be treated for 6 months in case of paucibacillary and 12 months in case of multibacillary. Further, precaution should be always taken to treat a confirmed disease, as many diseases mimic leprosy.

In closing, the authors highlight the current evidence about the association of vitamin D and VDR to leprosy disease progression. This knowledge will help in developing new strategies for the treatment and clinical management of leprosy patients.

Chapter 1 - Despite the availability of multidrug therapy since 1981, leprosy remains a significant public health problem and cause of disability in developing countries. Progress towards the control of leprosy has stagnated: over the last ten years, the global incidence has remained around 200,000 cases, 80% of which occur in India, Brazil, and Indonesia. Control efforts have been stymied by myriad factors, including stigma, which can delay diagnosis and treatment, as well as the paucity of information about where and to what extent transmission is occurring. These challenges are exacerbated by the lack of reliable data, the absence of an appropriate measure of leprosy burden, several gaps in the epidemiological knowledge about the disease, and the high cost of implementing new control measures. To accelerate progress towards a leprosy-free world, the World Health Organization (WHO) launched a global leprosy strategy in 2016 with the goal of achieving zero disability among new pediatric patients and reducing grade-2 disability rate to less than 1 case per 1 million people by 2020. To meet these goals, expanding knowledge about leprosy epidemiology, developing innovative, evidence-based strategies and optimal implementation of current programs are essential. In this chapter, the authors discuss the current public health challenges that leprosy control faces, and explore the opportunities addressing these challenges that can potentially accelerate progress towards the elimination of leprosy.

Chapter 2 - Leprosy is the least contagious of infectious diseases; it is caused by *M. leprae* and *M. lepromatosis* and mainly affects the skin and peripheral nerves. In addition to the existing interest because of the variation in the clinical characteristics of the disease between people, the immune response in this pathology will also differ; the way the immune system attacks the pathogen depends on the leprosy type that the patient exhibits. In general, the immune system is divided into 2 major branches: the innate immune system and the adaptive immune system. The innate immune system makes the first contact with the leprosy bacillus; it is composed of epithelial barriers, proteins with antimicrobial properties and cells such as neutrophils, macrophages, dendritic cells, NK, among others.

Most of these components exert their functions through several glycolipids recognition, that are found on the cell wall of *M. leprae,* by pattern recognition receptors (PRRs); among these are Toll-like receptors (TLR), with TLR2, TLR1/2 dimer, and TLR4 being the most important in the recognition of Hansen's bacillus. On the other hand, the adaptive immune system is composed of T lymphocytes ($CD4^+$ and $CD8^+$) and B lymphocytes. In turn, $CD4^+$ T cells are divided into different subpopulations (mainly Th1, Th2, Th17, Tregs) which are characterized by the production of different cytokine profiles. Patients with tuberculoid leprosy have an immune response mediated by Th1 cells, which is effective against intracellular bacteria and it is characterized by the production of IFN-γ, IL-12, and IL-2. In contrast, patients with lepromatous leprosy show a Th2 type immune response with the production of IL-4, IL-5, and IL-13. This profile is effective against extracellular parasites; therefore, it is ineffective against *M. leprae*, allowing its proliferation. In this chapter, the authors will review some immunological aspects of patients with leprosy and how this can be correlated with the clinical signs of the disease.

Chapter 3 - Leprosy is an infectious skin disease caused by *Mycobacterium leprae* (*M. leprae*). *M. leprae* can invade keratinocytes cells, macrophages cells, dendritic cells (DCs), and Schwann cells. *M. leprae* can induce various clinical manifestation depending on genetic susceptibility and the host immune system. The host immune system plays a vital role in leprosy pathogenesis. Leprosy patients can present as a broad spectrum of clinical manifestation, which are classified as paucibacillary (PB) type and multibacillary (MB) type. In the course of the disease, leprosy patients can experience episodes of acute inflammatory reactions known as leprosy reactions. Leprosy reactions are complications that may occur before, during, or after treatment, and cause further neurological damage that can cause chronic disabilities. This review will discuss the role of the immune response in leprosy pathogenesis and leprosy reactions.

Chapter 4 - The treatment of leprosy is always based on the final clinical and laboratory confirmation of the diagnosis. The diagnosed patient must be treated for 6 months in case of paucibacillary and 12 months in case of multibacillary Further, precaution should be always taken to treat a confirmed disease than by trial or error method, as many diseases mimic leprosy. At present three drugs, Rifampicin, Dapsone and clofazimine are given to multibacillary leprosy cases and two drugs, Rifampicin and Dapsone are given to paucibacillary leprosy cases. Both the cases are given drugs in Blister Calendar Packs (BCP). Recently, the World Health Organisation (WHO) has updated the guideline for the treatment of leprosy. The WHO has emphasized to use three drugs for 6 months and 12 months for the two types of leprosy paucibacillary and multibacillary, respectively. There is also a standard guideline to use certain regimen in case of individual drug relapse. In addition, chemoprophylaxis of contacts of confirmed leprosy cases have also been updated in the guideline. Besides the established drug regimine, there are also many alternate regimines followed in special cases of contraindication and due to adverse effects.In addition to the regular treatment regimine, the treatment of leprosy includes management of lepra reactions with Non Steroidal anti-Inflammatory Drugs (NSAIDS), steroids in needed cases, and clofazimine and thalidomide in special situation like erythema nodosum leprosum(ENL). Moreover, lots of immunosuppressants have also been tried in lepra reactions. All the aspects of the treatment will be detailed out throughout the chapters.

Chapter 5 - Leprosy or Hansen's disease is a re-emerging neglected tropical disease caused by *M. leprae*. Most of the leprosy cases have been reported from Indian subcontinent, several tropical countries in Africa and parts of Latin America. In 2017, nearly 200,000 new cases of leprosy were reported and highest prevalence was from India. Multidrug therapy (MDT), consisting of dapsone, rifampicin and clofazimine, is the current recommended treatment for leprosy. Most of the countries across the globe have eliminated leprosy (prevalence is <1 per 10,000). However, emergence of drug-resistant strains and relapse cases are of concern. Therefore, clinical management of leprosy needs implementation of new strategies. Leprosy is often termed as the 'disease of poor' as the disease is more prevalent among people living with insufficient food and shelter. Vitamin D is a micronutrient and its inadequate intake is associated with many types of health problems including decreased immunity against bacterial and viral infections. Several studies have indicated that vitamin D deficiency is associated with tuberculosis and HIV, though based on current evidences it is inconclusive to say that vitamin D deficiency is the risk factor for prevalence and severity of these diseases. Lower vitamin D level is thought to be associated with leprosy disease as vitamin D is a modulator of Th1, Th2 and toll-like receptor (TLR) signaling and these are the major immune response pathways against *M. leprae*. Also, the countries where vitamin D deficiency is prevalent, the number of leprosy cases is higher and more new cases are reported as compared to the other countries. Vitamin D acts through its receptor VDR, hence VDR is equally important in vitamin D mediated immunity. Recent reports concluded the linkage between low VDR expressions and risk of severe forms of leprosy disease, suggesting that vitamin D and VDR based therapy may be helpful in clinical management of infected individuals and prevent the emergence of new cases. In this chapter the authors have highlighted the current evidences about the association of vitamin D and VDR to leprosy disease progression, hinting more systematic studies is warranted to better understand the intrinsic pathways involved. The knowledge will help in developing new strategies for treatment and clinical management of leprosy patients.

In: Leprosy: From Diagnosis to Treatment ISBN: 978-1-53616-629-3
Editor: Daniel L. Knuth

Chapter 1

PUBLIC HEALTH CHALLENGES AND OPPORTUNITIES IN LEPROSY CONTROL: FROM THEORY TO IMPLEMENTATION

Sarah A. Galvani-Townsend, Pratha Sah, PhD and Abhishek Pandey*, PhD
Center for Infectious Disease Modeling and Analysis,
Yale School of Public Health, New Haven, CT, US

ABSTRACT

Despite the availability of multidrug therapy since 1981, leprosy remains a significant public health problem and cause of disability in developing countries. Progress towards the control of leprosy has stagnated: over the last ten years, the global incidence has remained around 200,000 cases, 80% of which occur in India, Brazil, and Indonesia. Control efforts have been stymied by myriad factors, including stigma, which can delay diagnosis and treatment, as well as the paucity of information about where and to what extent transmission is occurring. These challenges are exacerbated by the lack of reliable data, the absence of an appropriate measure of leprosy burden, several gaps in the epidemiological knowledge about the disease, and the high cost of

* Corresponding Author's E-mail: abhishek.pandey@yale.edu.

implementing new control measures. To accelerate progress towards a leprosy-free world, the World Health Organization (WHO) launched a global leprosy strategy in 2016 with the goal of achieving zero disability among new pediatric patients and reducing grade-2 disability rate to less than 1 case per 1 million people by 2020. To meet these goals, expanding knowledge about leprosy epidemiology, developing innovative, evidence-based strategies and optimal implementation of current programs are essential. In this chapter, we discuss the current public health challenges that leprosy control faces, and explore the opportunities addressing these challenges that can potentially accelerate progress towards the elimination of leprosy.

INTRODUCTION

Leprosy is an infectious disease caused by *Mycobacterium leprae* that primarily affects the skin and peripheral nerves. Primary symptoms of leprosy include muscle weakness, skin lesions, and numbness in the arms and legs. Although the mechanism of disease transmission is not known, it is generally accepted that prolonged, close contact with an untreated person is needed to catch the disease [1]. Clinical manifestation of leprosy infection appears after an incubation period ranging from 2 to 20 years [2]. Leprosy patients are divided into three groups based on the number of skin lesions and infected nerves involved: paucibacillary (PB) single-lesion leprosy (one skin lesion), paucibacillary leprosy (2-5 skin lesions) and multibacillary (MB) leprosy (more than five skin lesions) [3]. Symptoms of PB infection include swelling of the nerves, muscle weakness, numbness in the limbs and stuffy nose. Compared to PB leprosy, there are many outward symptoms associated with MB leprosy, including skin lesions, curling of the fingers, ulcers, and absorption of limbs. MB leprosy progresses at a rapid rate compared to PB leprosy, and patients with MB manifestation have a lower life expectancy. MB is also associated with greater life-long disability and has a higher transmission rate than PB. The immune responses and the mechanisms involved in nerve damage caused by leprosy are not well understood, and there is no predictive test to determine the extent of nerve damage as well as the best course of the treatment regimen to minimize the damage. The disabilities caused by leprosy are often irreversible [4]. Consequently, it is necessary to diagnose and treat leprosy infections early.

The first breakthrough of disease control occurred in 1941 when sulfone was introduced as a treatment for leprosy (Figure 1). Patients treated with sulfone were instructed to continue taking the drug in smaller doses after they were released from medical care. This was followed by dapsone in 1950 (Figure 1). Dapsone treatment typically continued for 4-10 years and, in some cases, treatment continued for life. However, *M. leprae* evolved resistance to dapsone in the 1960s, which reduced the effectiveness of dapsone. To combat this problem, multidrug therapy (MDT) was recommended by the World Health Organization (WHO) in 1981 (Figure 1). Current MDT treatment to cure single lesion paucibacillary leprosy includes a combination of rifampicin, ofloxacin, and minocycline. Paucibacillary leprosy is treated with a combination of Rifampicin and dapsone. A combination of Rifampicin, clofazimine, and dapsone is used to treat multibacillary leprosy [5].

Since 1995, the WHO has supplied MDT free of cost to leprosy patients in all endemic countries (Figure 1). MDT helped reduce worldwide prevalence from more than 5.25 million cases to approximately 193,118 since 1985 [6]. Global elimination of leprosy, defined as a registered prevalence of less than 1 case per 10,000 population, was achieved in 2000 [7]. Of the 122 countries previously considered endemic for leprosy, 119 countries had achieved leprosy elimination by 2012 [8]. This dramatic reduction in prevalence is almost entirely due to the shortening of treatment duration to two years. Following evidence of low relapse rates with MDT treatment for 24 months [9], the treatment duration was further reduced to a fixed period of 6 months for PB leprosy and 12 months for MB leprosy. Widespread use of MDT also reduced the long-term cost of treatment to the health system.

Despite the substantial progress made in the last 20 years, leprosy remains a significant public health problem and the leading cause of permanent physical disabilities due to a communicable disease [10]. More than 200,000 cases are still reported worldwide every year, with India, Brazil, and Indonesia accounting for 80% of the new cases detected globally [11]. While the global incidence of leprosy has declined by 3.4% over the last ten years, the increase in new cases was reported in 7 countries (Bangladesh, Brazil, Comoros, Mozambique, Nepal, Philippines and Sri Lanka) out of the 22 priority countries (Figure 2). Moreover, the number of new cases detected with grade-2 disability in 2017 only declined by 10% over the last 4 years from 12,267 to 11,014, indicating an urgent need to improve early case detection (Figure 3). Clearly, the transmission of leprosy is continuing. Eradication of leprosy will require increased efforts and a multifaceted strategy that addresses the myriad epidemiological, socioeconomic and clinical challenges that contribute to the persistence of leprosy. In this chapter, we review both pressing challenges and potential solutions to control leprosy.

KNOWLEDGE GAPS IN EPIDEMIOLOGY OF LEPROSY

An understanding of the transmission dynamics of leprosy is fundamental to the design and success of control strategies. However, there are gaps in our knowledge about the epidemiology of the disease. Firstly, the mechanism of leprosy transmission is not well understood. Leprosy is generally believed to spread either through direct exposure to infected fluids, indirectly via airborne viral droplets, or through direct or insect-mediated infection from zoonotic or environmental reservoirs [12]. Nasal secretions and skin of untreated leprosy patients are capable of shedding *M. leprae* to the environment. The relative potential of both the sites in establishing infection remains unclear. The ability of the disease to transmit over the course of an infection is also not known. Secondly, there is limited knowledge about risk factors for leprosy infection including genetic predisposition, immune and nutritional status [13]. Finally, there are the proportion of cases attributable to environmental reservoirs and animal hosts such as armadillos in the Americas [14, 15], red squirrels in the British Isles [16] and nonhuman primates [17].

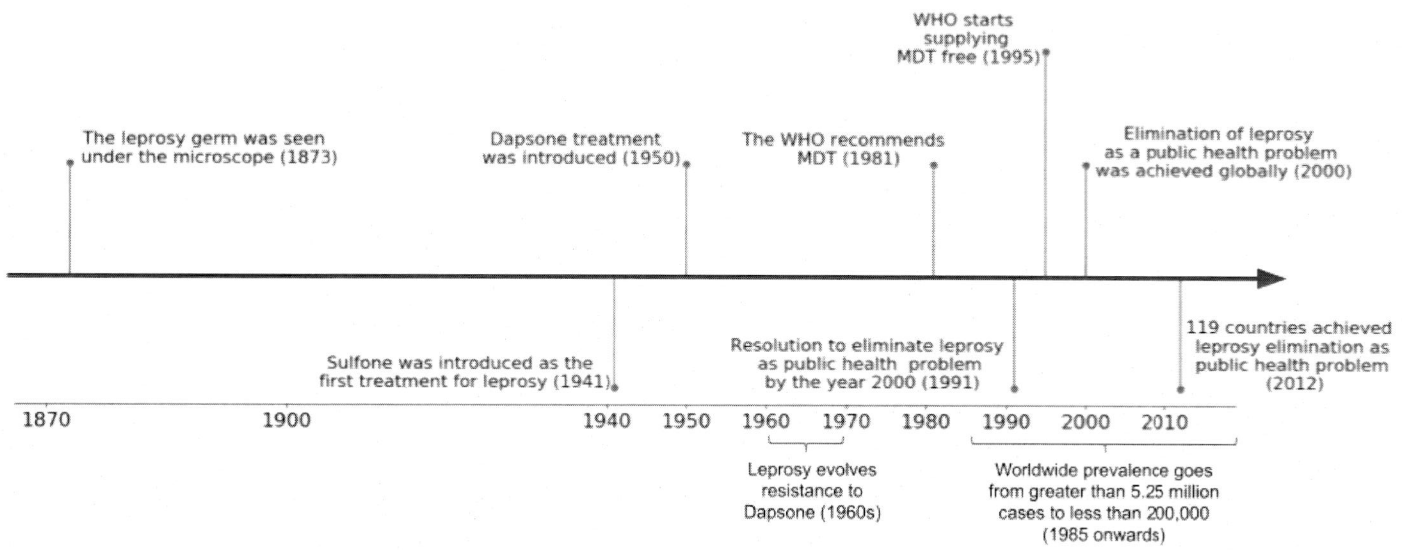

Figure 1. Timeline of key events in the history of leprosy.

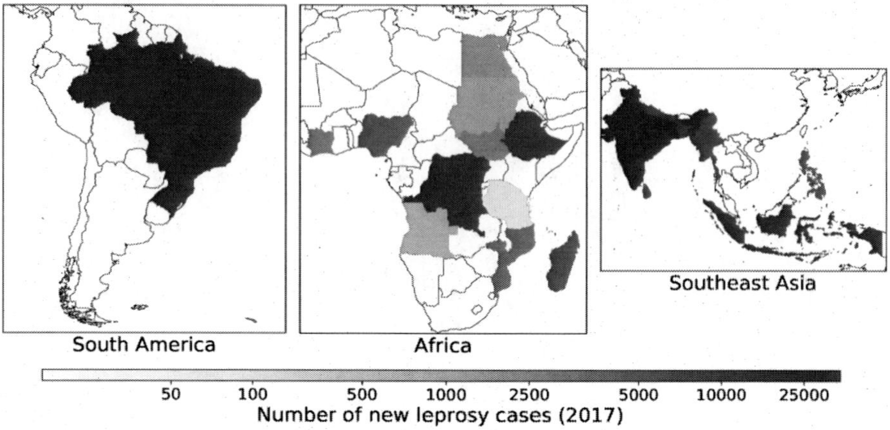

Figure 2. Number of new leprosy cases across the 22 global priority countries in 2017.

A better understanding of *M. leprae* transmission, as well as the risk factors for infection, is essential to developing effective interventions to interrupt transmission. While the mode of leprosy transmission is unclear, prolonged, close contact with an untreated patient is likely the most common cause of transmission. Contact tracing, which involves reaching out to the contacts of index patients and screening them for signs of leprosy, can be an effective strategy of curbing leprosy transmission by enabling early diagnosis and identifying additional cases [18–21]. Research focusing on the relationship between human genetics and *M. leprae* genome has been crucial towards developing an understanding of how and why people develop leprosy [22]. There have been an increasing number of reports linking genetic regulation of the innate immune response with increased susceptibility to leprosy and also to the development of adverse leprosy reactions [23]. Advanced genome-wide association studies have provided clues towards immune-related gene variants that pose as risk factors for leprosy [24–27].

CHOOSING A METRIC TO MONITOR LEPROSY CONTROL

An appropriate definition of leprosy control is fundamental to optimize strategic interventions, setting geographical priorities, and estimate the impact of intervention efforts. Prevalence has been one of the most widely used measures of monitoring leprosy burden and control. However, disease prevalence is a poor indicator of leprosy control because it is sensitive to factors such as incubation period of the disease, duration of treatment and case-finding method [28, 29]. Firstly, leprosy has a long incubation period, ranging from 2 to 20 years [30], and technology to detect leprosy at early stage is lacking. New cases therefore continue to become infectious even if prevalence may have been very low in a particular year. Secondly, with MDT, patients are declared cured after treatment and removed from leprosy registers. Consequently, shortening the treatment duration alone can dramatically reduced prevalence without reducing the number of new cases detected annually. For example, the global burden of registered leprosy cases reduced by 50% when the treatment period of leprosy decreased from 24 months to 12 months [31]. Besides prevalence, new case detection rate is increasingly used to report leprosy burden across the world. Both prevalence and new case detection rates suffer as a metric by the fact that they are strongly dependent on the surveillance efforts. Furthermore, as countries are not required to provide evidence of the quality and effectiveness of surveillance efforts, levels of under-reporting remain uncertain.

Challenges in choosing a metric to monitor leprosy control can be overcome by adopting several indicators rather than a single one. Case detection among children provides good evidence for ongoing active transmission of leprosy, and therefore new case reports among children along with disease prevalence data and detection rate can be utilized to better monitor the ongoing transmission as well as inform intervention approaches [32, 33]. Previous modeling studies have highlighted the need for active case detection [34, 35]. Such mathematical models of leprosy transmission can be further utilized to understand the current and future disease burden based on historical data and scientific knowledge about the disease. Moreover, such studies can allow us to assess the impact of under-reporting and evaluate the effectiveness of current and future intervention strategies to curtail transmission.

SETTING A GLOBAL TARGET FOR LEPROSY CONTROL

In 1991, the WHO defined the goal of eliminating leprosy as reducing the global prevalence rate to less than one case per 10,000 population. Although the global goal was achieved in 2000, India and Brazil failed to meet the deadline. The deadline was extended to 2005 for both India and Brazil that lead to some unintended consequences. For example, India began relying on voluntary reporting and stopped actively seeking new cases and screening contacts. As a result, detection rates fell by 75% between 2003 and 2005 [36]. In India, almost half of the cases were not reported or were staged inappropriately as part of an effort to formally meet the elimination targets of 2005 [37]. Similarly, Brazil achieved the target in 2005 when unregistered patients were omitted from the calculation, which was later retracted after the missing patients were reinstated [36]. The quality of the reported data still remains a concern, especially from low-income countries. The poorest areas tend to have longer detection delays that result in larger numbers of undiagnosed leprosy cases. These undiagnosed cases remain a critical threat to the goal of breaking transmission. When countries are pressured to eliminate leprosy, inaccurate reports can ensue in an attempt to pretend to meet the goal. A study estimated that over 2.6 million cases were missed between 2000 and 2012 due to the decline in new case detection rates for meeting the Leprosy elimination target [37]. Inaccurate and under-reporting of cases not only result in continued transmission and delays in starting treatment, but also a shortage of drugs required for treatment. Therefore, it is essential to ensure that leprosy goals are transparent and widely understandable.

Setting an inappropriate global target of control can also mislead governments, health workers and donors. For example, following the achievement of previous elimination goal in 2000, political commitment, funding, and training of healthcare workers lost momentum, even though more than 700,000 new cases were registered in the same year [10, 36, 38]. The decreased incentive to find new cases may partly explain the 38% increase in grade-2 disability cases from 2004 - 2007. Recognizing these challenges and shortcomings of defining goals based on elimination, the WHO shifted its future goal towards reducing the global burden and reduction of grade-2 disabilities. The 2016-2020 Global Leprosy Strategy aims to reduce the newly detected cases with leprosy-related deformities to below 1 per million population at the global level by 2020 and to reduce leprosy-affected disabilities in children to zero. The WHO's new goal of reducing the grade-2 disability rate will be challenging, considering uncertainties about data quality. Tools and measurement techniques for collecting disability data exist, but their applicability to leprosy-endemic countries needs to be validated [39].

CLINICAL SHORTCOMINGS

Currently, the evidence of acid-fast bacilli in slit-skin smears or the presence of characteristic histological patterns of nerves or skin through biopsy is used to confirm a diagnosis of leprosy. However, the presence of bacilli is rare in the PB forms of the disease and in some cases typical histopathologic changes may not be present [40]. Therefore, there is no gold standard for accurately diagnosing and classifying leprosy so far. Moreover, there are no serologic tests that are available for the routine laboratory diagnosis.

In the absence of any point-of-care test, the initial diagnosis of leprosy commonly relies on the patient's clinical signs and symptoms. In an endemic area, WHO recommends considering an individual as having leprosy if they have skin lesions consistent with definite sensory loss, with or without thickened nerves and positive skin smears. The clinical symptoms are determined by a skin and neurological exam. Additionally, skin biopsies and smears may also be taken to provide a more conclusive diagnosis. Other more uncommon tests include nasal smears, nerve biopsies, and blood exams. Based on the number of bacteria, either PB or MB leprosy is diagnosed [41].

Since leprosy patients have traditionally been in the hands of specialized staff, many healthcare providers are ill-equipped to treat leprosy patients. Success in meeting the World Health Organization's (WHO) goal of eliminating leprosy as a global public health problem by 2005 also led to complacency and a loss of skills in diagnosing and managing leprosy patients. Although the integration of leprosy services into public health services helps reduce stigma, there is a loss of skill in diagnosis and treatment. [42]. Lack of diagnosis and management skills is exacerbated by the fact that, even if a clinical diagnosis is made, there is no good point-of-care test for confirming it. [43]. Tests to confirm a leprosy diagnosis such as skin smears and skin biopsies are only available in facilities that have labs. Unavailability of such facilities can also lead to patients being diagnosed with a disease other than leprosy by their healthcare providers. 42.6% of participants in a study among patients across three states of Brazil were misdiagnosed initially, suggesting a need to increase clinical suspicion of leprosy [44].

In order to both curb transmission and prevent disabilities, it is essential to focus on research aimed at finding practical diagnostic tools that can detect all levels of leprosy infections. Several serological tests for leprosy detection are under development but none of them have achieved sufficient sensitivity and specificity yet [42]. Integrating leprosy services in primary health care can improve case finding and continuity of care, however without appropriate expertise, misdiagnosis of leprosy can not be minimized. Therefore, it is vital to provide clinicians training to recognize and diagnose leprosy, especially in high-risk regions.

STIGMA OF LEPROSY

Although leprosy has had a widespread prevalence since medieval times, and there is evidence of the disease as far back as 1600 BC, it was not until 1873 that *M. leprae* was discovered as the cause of leprosy. While this discovery dispelled the myth that leprosy was hereditary or a curse, the stigma associated with the disease persisted. Fuelling the stigma, legal discrimination against people affected by leprosy played a key role in outcasting leprosy patients from society. For example, segregation of people with leprosy was required by law in Japan and leprosy patients begged for a living around the temples or shrines. Starting in 1909, the Japanese government started hospitalizing leprosy patients in the leprosy sanatoria, often forcefully. This law lasted until 1996 [45]. Similarly, British India enacted the Leprosy Act of 1898, which institutionalized those affected and segregated them by sex to prevent reproduction. The law also stated that a state government could declare any place as an asylum for people with leprosy. In addition, a sequel to the law said that any person with leprosy who appeared to be poor could be arrested without a warrant. This law was repealed only in 1983 [46].

Although legal discrimination against leprosy patients has reduced significantly across the world, the social stigma against people with leprosy continues to drive affected individuals into further poverty by limiting their employment and educational opportunities. Because MB leprosy shows more outward signs of the disease, people with MB leprosy are stigmatized more than people with PB leprosy. Stigma also deters people from seeking treatment that subsequently leads to irreversible disabilities, such as nerve damage [42]. Delayed treatment also increases the risk of transmission to other people. While active case finding can curb transmission in areas where stigma is widespread, efforts to reduce social stigma towards leprosy patients will have a long-lasting impact on surveillance and control of leprosy.

The stigma associated with the disease is deeply rooted in societies across the world through centuries of misconceptions and myths. The lack of knowledge about the etiology, curability, and transmissibility of the disease remains one of the driving factors of social stigma faced by leprosy patients. Therefore, interventions to raise community awareness by demystifying misconceptions such as leprosy being hereditary or leprosy cases being untouchable can be highly effective. Similarly, it is imperative to train healthcare officials and staff to ensure non-discriminatory behavior of healthcare workers while diagnosing and treating leprosy patients. Integrating leprosy services in general health care aimed towards 'no isolation-no discrimination' policy can gradually decrease society's negative perception as well as provide treatment to leprosy patients closer home.

Fear of social exclusion plays a fundamental role in leprosy patients delaying seeking treatment. The deformity caused by leprosy in a patient not only limits their employment opportunities, but it also results in decreased prospects of marriage for them and their family members. Strategies that primarily focus on reintegration of people with leprosy into society such that they can live with dignity and self-sufficiency are essential to improve their quality of life and to encourage individuals with symptoms to seek early treatment.

The WHO's Global Leprosy Strategy 2016-2020 calls for several measures to end discrimination towards those affected by leprosy [47]. These measures include empowering the leprosy patients and their communities to actively participate in leprosy programs, providing better access to social and financial support, and promoting community-based rehabilitation for people with leprosy-related disabilities. The WHO has also committed to work towards ending discriminatory laws and promoting policies that facilitate the inclusion of people affected by leprosy.

Socioeconomic Risk Factors

Although leprosy has been identified as a disease of poverty, we still have a limited understanding of the risk factors that link them together. Nationally, new case detection rates do not necessarily correlate with indicators such as GDP or human development index. For example, countries with very low human development index such as Burkina Faso (ranked 183) and Benin (ranked 163) report lower new case detection rates compared to Brazil (ranked 79) that has the second highest new case detection rates [48]. The distribution of leprosy risk is highly heterogeneous even within most affected countries such as India, Brazil and Indonesia where the majority of cases occur in high-risk regions. Living in a crowded household as well as lack of schooling was identified as a risk factor in an individual-level study done in Malawi [49]. Another study conducted in a high endemic area of leprosy in Brazil showed the level of inequality, population growth, and presence of a railroad are associated with higher levels of leprosy [50]. A systematic review and meta-analysis of 39 studies identified poor hygiene, lower levels of education, and food insecurity as risk factors for leprosy [51].

Across all high-endemic regions of leprosy, impoverished communities remain disproportionately affected. Multiple socioeconomic factors drive the association between leprosy and poverty. One of these factors is the lack of physical access to diagnosis and treatment, which occurs due to inadequate access to specialized leprosy clinics. The costs of seeking treatment are another factor. Although MDT is free, other costs such as travel, lost wages, and other incidental expenses must be accounted for. In addition, getting MDT to patients—who are typically located in impoverished remote locations—poses major logistical and distribution challenges. Shortages of MDT at the health center level are a chronic problem due to weak information systems and inadequate planning. Moreover, when the disease has progressed too far, MDT may not be sufficient to prevent permanent disabilities.

Most of these challenges emphasize the importance of efficient, cost-effective case detection in high-endemic regions. The status quo approach of passive case finding that relies on people with symptoms to voluntarily present themselves at health-care facilities is ill-suited to curb transmission. Delayed treatment also increases the risk of permanent disabilities. Targeted strategies of diagnosing cases in high-risk areas have the potential to accelerate leprosy control. By facilitating early diagnosis and treatment, targeted case-finding approaches can substantially curtail transmission and reduce disabilities among leprosy patients. Socioeconomic factors associated with high risk can of leprosy infection be used to target diagnostic efforts and interventions that will be fundamental to curb leprosy transmission. Moreover, improving health-care access and implementing poverty alleviating interventions among the most vulnerable populations in leprosy-endemic regions can facilitate leprosy control.

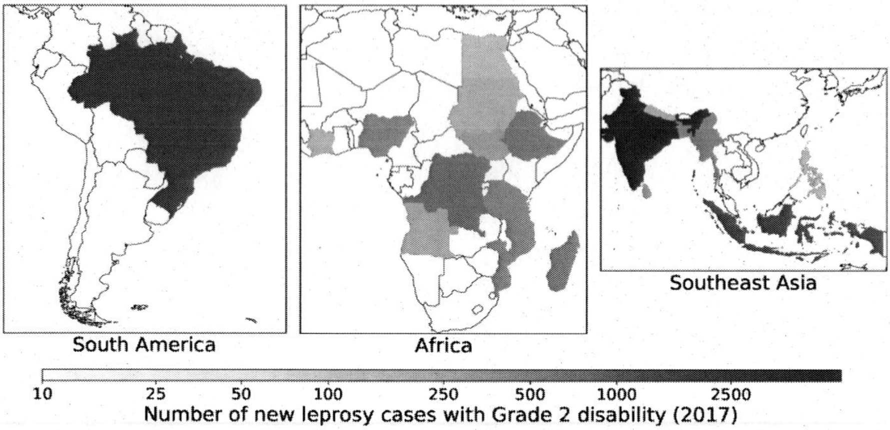

Figure 3. Number of new leprosy cases diagnosed with grade-2 disabilities across the 22 global priority countries in 2017.

CONCLUSION

Leprosy, an age-old disease caused by *Mycobacterium leprae*, is no longer causing the level of devastation it had for thousands of years. Since multidrug therapy became available for widespread use in the early 1980s, over 16 million people have been successfully treated for leprosy [52]. Consequently, leprosy prevalence has dropped by 99% over the last thirty years: from 21.1 cases per 10,000 population in 1985 to 0.2 cases per 10,000 population in 2015 [52]. Progress towards leprosy control, however, has stagnated due to continuing and interrelated challenges of clinical uncertainties, knowledge gaps in epidemiology of leprosy, stigma, delayed diagnosis, and socioeconomic risk factors [53].

A multifaceted approach that mitigates the existing challenges and improves early case-detection, provides effective treatment and reintegrates leprosy patients in the society will be required to curtail leprosy at local and global levels. It is vital to identify the pockets of high endemicity in each country. Intervention efforts can be most effectively and efficiently targeted to these areas where high-risk population reside. Innovative technologies are needed to generate high quality and high-resolution data on new case detection rates and prevalence. Epidemiological studies can utilize these data to identify factors that are associated with a high risk of leprosy and to map the regions where control efforts are most needed. For example, a recent systematic review and meta-analysis of socioeconomic determinants revealed several risk factors, including crowded living conditions, food insecurity, household exposure, manual labor, increasing age, lack of sanitation, and lower levels of education [51].

Untrained healthcare professionals contribute substantially to delays in case detection due to both misdiagnoses of early-stage symptoms and discriminatory behavior towards leprosy patients. Training and sensitizing healthcare workers to create a nondiscriminatory healthcare environment will reduce misdiagnosis of cases and encourage patients with symptoms to seek treatment sooner. Delays in diagnosis can also be reduced by alleviating the social stigma faced by patients. Awareness campaigns can aid in reducing societal stigma and contribute to accelerating case-detection and preventing leprosy-related deformities in patients. In the absence of quick point-of-care tests for confirming leprosy, setting up a sufficient number of laboratories with facilities to conduct skin and nerve biopsy and acid-bacilli tests can also improve case-detection rates. Given that leprosy is a disease of poverty, social development should help to reduce leprosy risks and facilitate eradication.

As leprosy has a very long incubation period, rigorous surveillance and contact tracing are of utmost importance to curb transmission in communities where leprosy cases have been reported. The WHO recommends examining the members of a patient's household for signs of leprosy and educating them on the initial signs. The approach can be further strengthened by continued periodic inspections of family members by medical professionals. At the community level, active case finding should be implemented in areas from leprosy cases are being reported. Awareness campaigns can educate communities to recognize the first signs of symptoms so that they can seek medical care promptly before permanent disabilities occur or there is a further onward transmission. In areas that have previously reported cases, surveillance can be implemented via periodic active case finding among school children to monitor leprosy transmission. The government of countries with leprosy should frame health policies that are geared towards reducing transmission.

The treatment-as-prevention approaches that have been successful in curtailing HIV transmission are applicable to leprosy. Chemoprophylaxis, a treatment that prevents infection for about two years, is an option that can significantly lower the risk of leprosy acquisition among contacts of leprosy patients. However, the widespread use of chemoprophylaxis is still being debated due to ethical and logistical concerns [42, 54]. Two doses of chemoprophylaxis, as opposed to one, would be most effective, but chemoprophylaxis is expensive and is not widely available [54]. Cost-effectiveness studies can evaluate and optimize strategies to treat and household contacts of leprosy patients using chemoprophylaxis. Furthermore, the Bacillus Calmette–Guérin (BCG) vaccine, which provides protection against tuberculosis, has also been found to be partially efficacious against leprosy [55]. Thus, BCG vaccination coverage levels should be assessed among populations that are at high risk of leprosy. Improving BCG vaccination among individuals at high risk of leprosy can be a cost-effective strategy for averting cases of leprosy and ultimately reducing prevalence.

Following the introduction of MDT, leprosy prevalence declined sharply between 1980 to 2010. The positive impact of widespread use of MDT appears to have run its course and despite continued efforts, leprosy prevalence has remained stable for the last several years. There is a need for new innovative tools that can detect leprosy infection early, including subclinical infection, and tracking drug resistance. Additionally, new avenues for basic science and clinical research have been opened by genome sequencing of *Mycobacterium leprae* and genome-wide analysis for leprosy cases, which could be instrumental in the development of drugs and vaccines. Until such breakthroughs in clinical research are achieved that can augment the current strategies and facilitate the elimination of leprosy, interrupting leprosy transmission will require bolstering skills in leprosy diagnosis and management, rigorous surveillance and contact tracing of cases, and development of a point-of-care test for confirming leprosy diagnosis.

REFERENCES

[1] Transmission | *Hansen's Disease (Leprosy)* | CDC [Internet]. 15 Jan 2019 [cited 6 Sep 2019]. Available: https://www.cdc.gov/leprosy/transmission/index.html

[2] *Leprosy* [Internet]. [cited 17 Sep 2019]. Available: https://www.who.int/en/news-room/fact-sheets/detail/leprosy.

[3] *WHO Model Prescribing Information: Drugs Used in Leprosy: Classification of leprosy* [Internet]. [cited 5 Sep 2019]. Available: https://apps.who.int/medicinedocs/en/d/Jh2988e/4.html.

[4] Geluk, A. Correlates of immune exacerbations in leprosy. *Semin Immunol.*, 2018, 39, 111–118.

[5] *WHO Model Prescribing Information: Drugs Used in Leprosy: Treatment of leprosy* [Internet]. [cited 5 Sep 2019]. Available: https://apps.who.int/medicinedocs/en/d/Jh2988e/5.html.

[6] International Textbook of Leprosy. In: *International Textbook of Leprosy* [Internet]. [cited 17 Sep 2019]. Available: https://internationaltextbookofleprosy.org/.

[7] *Leprosy* [Internet]. [cited 4 Jun 2019]. Available: https://www.who.int/news-room/fact-sheets/detail/leprosy.

[8] World Health Organization. Accelerating work to overcome the global impact of neglected tropical diseases: a roadmap for implementation. Executive summary. *World Health Organization Geneva*, 2012.

[9] Ji, B. Why multidrug therapy for multibacillary leprosy can be shortened to 12 months. *Lepr Rev.*, 1998, 69, 106–109.

[10] Chaptini, C; Marshman, G. Leprosy: a review on elimination, reducing the disease burden, and future research. *Lepr Rev.*, 2015, 86, 307–315.

[11] *Global leprosy update, 2017: reducing the disease burden due to leprosy* [Internet]. World Health Organization; 2018 Aug. Available: https://apps.who.int/iris/bitstream/handle/10665/274289/WER9335.pdf.

[12] Bratschi, MW; Steinmann, P; Wickenden, A; Gillis, TP. Current knowledge on Mycobacterium leprae transmission: a systematic literature review. *Lepr Rev.*, 2015, 86, 142–155.

[13] Feenstra, SG; Nahar, Q; Pahan, D; Oskam, L; Richardus, JH. Recent food shortage is associated with leprosy disease in Bangladesh: a case-control study. *PLoS Negl Trop Dis.*, 2011, 5, e1029.

[14] Truman, RW; Singh, P; Sharma, R; Busso, P; Rougemont, J; Paniz-Mondolfi, A; et al. Probable zoonotic leprosy in the southern United States. *N Engl J Med.*, 2011, 364, 1626–1633.

[15] da Silva, MB; Portela, JM; Li, W; Jackson, M; Gonzalez-Juarrero, M; Hidalgo, AS; et al. Evidence of zoonotic leprosy in Pará, Brazilian Amazon, and risks associated with human contact or consumption of armadillos. *PLoS Negl Trop Dis.*, 2018, 12, e0006532.

[16] Avanzi, C; Del-Pozo, J; Benjak, A; Stevenson, K; Simpson, VR; Busso, P; et al. Red squirrels in the British Isles are infected with leprosy bacilli. *Science.*, 2016, 354, 744–747.

[17] Honap, TP; Pfister, LA; Housman, G; Mills, S; Tarara, RP; Suzuki, K; et al. Mycobacterium leprae genomes from naturally infected nonhuman primates. *PLoS Negl Trop Dis.*, 2018, 12, e0006190.

[18] Moet, FJ; Pahan, D; Schuring, RP; Oskam, L; Richardus, JH. Physical distance, genetic relationship, age, and leprosy classification are independent risk factors for leprosy in contacts of patients with leprosy. *J Infect Dis.*, 2006, 193, 346–353.

[19] Smith, WCS; Aerts, A. Role of contact tracing and prevention strategies in the interruption of leprosy transmission. *Lepr Rev.*, 2014, 85, 2–17.

[20] Barth-Jaeggi, T; Steinmann, P; Mieras, L; van Brakel, W; Richardus, JH; Tiwari, A; et al. Leprosy Post-Exposure Prophylaxis (LPEP) programme: study protocol for evaluating the feasibility and impact on case detection rates of contact tracing and single dose rifampicin. *BMJ Open.*, 2016, 6, e013633.

[21] Hacker, M de A; Duppre, NC; Nery, JAC; Sales, AM; Sarno, EN. Characteristics of leprosy diagnosed through the surveillance of contacts: a comparison with index cases in Rio de Janeiro, 1987-2010. *Mem Inst Oswaldo Cruz.*, 2012, 107, Suppl 1, 49–54.

[22] Sauer, MED; Salomão, H; Ramos, GB; D'Espindula, HRS; Rodrigues, RSA; Macedo, WC; et al. Genetics of leprosy: Expected- and unexpected-developments and perspectives. *Clin Dermatol.*, 2016, 34, 96–104.

[23] Polycarpou, A; Walker, SL; Lockwood, DN. New findings in the pathogenesis of leprosy and implications for the management of leprosy. *Curr Opin Infect Dis.*, 2013, 26, 413–419.

[24] Cambri, G; Mira, MT. Genetic Susceptibility to Leprosy-From Classic Immune-Related Candidate Genes to Hypothesis-Free, Whole Genome Approaches. *Front Immunol.*, 2018, 9, 1674.

[25] Siddiqui, MR; Meisner, S; Tosh, K; Balakrishnan, K; Ghei, S; Fisher, SE; et al. A major susceptibility locus for leprosy in India maps to chromosome 10p13. *Nat Genet.*, 2001, 27, 439–441.

[26] Tosh, K; Meisner, S; Siddiqui, MR; Balakrishnan, K; Ghei, S; Golding, M; et al. A region of chromosome 20 is linked to leprosy susceptibility in a South Indian population. *J Infect Dis.*, 2002, 186, 1190–1193.

[27] Wallace, C; Fitness, J; Hennig, B; Sichali, L; Mwaungulu, L; Pönnighaus, JM; et al. Linkage analysis of susceptibility to leprosy type using an IBD regression method. *Genes Immun.*, 2004, 5, 221–225.

[28] Durrheim, DN; Speare, R. Global leprosy elimination: time to change more than the elimination target date. *J Epidemiol Community Health.*, 2003, 57, 316–317.

[29] Smith, C; Richardus, JH. Leprosy strategy is about control, not eradication. *Lancet.*, 2008, 371, 969–970.

[30] *Leprosy* [Internet]. [cited 16 Sep 2019]. Available: https://www.who.int/en/news-room/fact-sheets/detail/leprosy.

[31] Prasad, PSS and Kaviarasan, PK. Leprosy therapy, past and present: can we hope to eliminate it? *Indian J Dermatol.*, 2010, 55, 316.

[32] Ezenduka, C; Post, E; John, S; Suraj, A; Namadi, A; Onwujekwe, O. Cost-effectiveness analysis of three leprosy case detection methods in Northern Nigeria. *PLoS Negl Trop Dis.*, 2012, 6, e1818.

[33] Pedrosa, VL; Dias, LC; Galban, E; Leturiondo, A; Palheta, J; Jr. Santos, M; et al. Leprosy among schoolchildren in the Amazon region: A cross-sectional study of active search and possible source of infection by contact tracing. *PLoS Negl Trop Dis.*, 2018, 12, e0006261.

[34] Blok, DJ; de Vlas, SJ; Fischer, EAJ; Richardus, JH. Chapter Two - Mathematical Modelling of Leprosy and Its Control. In: Anderson RM, Basáñez MG, editors. *Advances in Parasitology*. Academic Press, 2015, pp. 33–51.

[35] Blok, DJ; Crump, RE; Sundaresh, R; Ndeffo-Mbah, M; Galvani, AP; Porco, TC; et al. Forecasting the new case detection rate of leprosy in four states of Brazil: A comparison of modelling approaches [Internet]. *Epidemics.*, 2017, pp. 92–100. doi:10.1016/ j.epidem. 2017.01.005.

[36] Lockwood, DNJ; Shetty, V; Penna, GO. Hazards of setting targets to eliminate disease: lessons from the leprosy elimination campaign. *BMJ.*, 2014, 348, g1136.

[37] Blok, DJ; De Vlas, SJ; Richardus, JH. Global elimination of leprosy by 2020: are we on track? *Parasit Vectors.*, 2015, 8, 548.

[38] Lockwood, DNJ. Leprosy elimination-a virtual phenomenon or a reality? *BMJ.*, 2002, 324, 1516–1518.

[39] Van Brakel, WH; Officer, A. Approaches and tools for measuring disability in low and middle-income countries. *Lepr Rev.*, 2008, 79, 50–64.

[40] Scollard, DM; Adams, LB; Gillis, TP; Krahenbuhl, JL; Truman, RW; Williams, DL. The continuing challenges of leprosy. *Clin Microbiol Rev.*, 2006, 19, 338–381.

[41] Doerr, S. Leprosy: History, Symptoms and Treatment. In: *eMedicineHealth* [Internet]. [cited 8 Sep 2019]. Available: https://www.emedicinehealth.com/leprosy/article_em.htm.

[42] Rodrigues, LC; Lockwood, DN. Leprosy now: epidemiology, progress, challenges, and research gaps. *Lancet Infect Dis.*, 2011, 11, 464–470.

[43] Tatipally, S; Srikantam, A; Kasetty, S. Polymerase Chain Reaction (PCR) as a Potential Point of Care Laboratory Test for Leprosy Diagnosis—A Systematic Review. *Tropical Medicine and Infectious Disease.*, 2018, 3. doi:10.3390/tropicalmed3040107.

[44] Henry, M; GalAn, N; Teasdale, K; Prado, R; Amar, H; Rays, MS; et al. Factors Contributing to the Delay in Diagnosis and Continued Transmission of Leprosy in Brazil--An Explorative, Quantitative, Questionnaire Based Study. *PLoS Negl Trop Dis.*, 2016, 10, e0004542.

[45] Sato, H; Narita, M. Politics of leprosy segregation in Japan: the emergence, transformation and abolition of the patient segregation policy. *Soc Sci Med.*, 2003, 56, 2529–2539.

[46] *India's repeal of 1898 Lepers Act is small step but giant leaps remain* | News | News & resources | The Leprosy Mission [Internet]. [cited 17 Sep 2019]. Available: https://www.leprosymission.org.uk/news-and-resources/news/indias-repeal-of-1898-lepers-act-is-positive-step/.

[47] Regional Office for South-East Asia, World Health Organization. *Global Leprosy Strategy 2016-2020: Accelerating towards a leprosy-free world.* WHO Regional Office for South-East Asia, 2016.

[48] Lockwood, DNJ. Commentary: leprosy and poverty. *International journal of epidemiology.*, 2004, pp. 269–270.

[49] Ponnighaus, JM; Fine, PE; Sterne, JA; Malema, SS; Bliss, L; Wilson, RJ. Extended schooling and good housing conditions are associated

with reduced risk of leprosy in rural Malawi. *Int J Lepr Other Mycobact Dis.*, 1994, 62, 345–352.

[50] Kerr-Pontes, LRS; Montenegro, ACD; Barreto, ML; Werneck, GL; Feldmeier, H. Inequality and leprosy in Northeast Brazil: an ecological study. *Int J Epidemiol.*, 2004, 33, 262–269.

[51] Pescarini, JM; Strina, A; Nery, JS; Skalinski, LM; Andrade, KVF; de, Penna, MLF; et al. Socioeconomic risk markers of leprosy in high-burden countries: A systematic review and meta-analysis. *PLoS Negl Trop Dis.*, 2018, 12, e0006622.

[52] World Health Organization, *Leprosy fact sheet.* 2017; Available: http://www.searo.who.int/entity/global_leprosy_programme/topics/factsheet/en/.

[53] Forno, C; Häusermann, P; Hatz, C; Itin, P; Blum, J. The Difficulty in Diagnosis and Treatment of Leprosy. *J Travel Med.*, 2010, 17, 281–283.

[54] Smith, CS; Noordeen, SK; Richardus, JH; Sansarricq, H; Cole, ST; Soares, RC; et al. A strategy to halt leprosy transmission. *Lancet Infect Dis.*, 2014, 14, 96–98.

[55] Merle, CSC; Cunha, SS; Rodrigues, LC. BCG vaccination and leprosy protection: review of current evidence and status of BCG in leprosy control. *Expert Rev Vaccines.*, 2010, 9, 209–222.

In: Leprosy: From Diagnosis to Treatment ISBN: 978-1-53616-629-3
Editor: Daniel L. Knuth

Chapter 2

LEPROSY IMMUNOLOGY

Mary Fafutis-Morris[1,*], PhD.
and Jorge J. R. Padilla-Arellano[2]
[1]Departamento de Fisiología, Universidad de Guadalajara
Guadalajara, Jalisco, Mexico
[2]Doctorado en Cs Biomédicas, Universidad de Guadalajara,
Guadalajara, Jalisco, Mexico

ABSTRACT

Leprosy is the least contagious of infectious diseases; it is caused by *M. leprae* and *M. lepromatosis* and mainly affects the skin and peripheral nerves. In addition to the existing interest because of the variation in the clinical characteristics of the disease between people, the immune response in this pathology will also differ; the way the immune system attacks the pathogen depends on the leprosy type that the patient exhibits.

In general, the immune system is divided into 2 major branches: the innate immune system and the adaptive immune system. The innate immune system makes the first contact with the leprosy bacillus; it is composed of epithelial barriers, proteins with antimicrobial properties and cells such as neutrophils, macrophages, dendritic cells, NK, among others. Most of these components exert their functions through several

* Corresponding Author's E-mail: mfafutis@gmail.com.

glycolipids recognition, that are found on the cell wall of *M. leprae,* by pattern recognition receptors (PRRs); among these are Toll-like receptors (TLR), with TLR2, TLR1/2 dimer, and TLR4 being the most important in the recognition of Hansen's bacillus.

On the other hand, the adaptive immune system is composed of T lymphocytes ($CD4^+$ and $CD8^+$) and B lymphocytes. In turn, $CD4^+$ T cells are divided into different subpopulations (mainly Th1, Th2, Th17, Tregs) which are characterized by the production of different cytokine profiles. Patients with tuberculoid leprosy have an immune response mediated by Th1 cells, which is effective against intracellular bacteria and it is characterized by the production of IFN-γ, IL-12, and IL-2. In contrast, patients with lepromatous leprosy show a Th2 type immune response with the production of IL-4, IL-5, and IL-13. This profile is effective against extracellular parasites; therefore, it is ineffective against *M. leprae*, allowing its proliferation.

In this chapter, we will review some immunological aspects of patients with leprosy and how this can be correlated with the clinical signs of the disease.

Leprosy Immunology

Leprosy, or Hansen's disease, represents the best natural biological model to study the immune response. This is due to its presentation along a spectrum, in which we find two stable poles that represent two T lymphocyte subpopulations and an intermediate continuum able to migrate to either of the two Th1/Th2 poles, depending on multiple factors. The aetiologic agents, *M. leprae* and the recently described *M. lepromatosis*, are obligate intracellular pathogens that cannot be cultured to date [1].

In this chapter we look at the leprosy immune response caused by *M. leprae*, since there is no information about *M. lepromatosis* so far.

Innate Immunity

The immune system cells that make the first contact with both mycobacteria belong to the innate immunity. These cells contain a variety of pattern recognition receptors (PRRs) that can be classified as RLRs,

NLRs, and TLRs. TLRs are a family of 10 receptors (in mammals) that are expressed in different immune system cells, as well as in epithelial cells [2].

TLR activation contributes to the innate immune response through the initiation of phagocytosis, the liberation of antimicrobial peptides, the induction and liberation of cytokines and chemokines, and the maturation of immune cells such as dendritic cells, which are critically important since they are the bridge between the innate and the adaptive immune response [3].

The cell wall of *M. leprae* is composed primarily of glycolipids, glycosylated phospholipids and complex carbohydrates linked to mycolic acid or peptides. The recognition of these diverse components through TLRs is a key step in the generation of the immune response against the infection. Each TLR can interact with specific bacterial molecules and against mycobacteria; TLR1, TLR2, TLR4 and the dimer TLR2/1 are the most important [4].

M. leprae activates mainly the TLR2 and the dimer TLR2/1, which indicates the presence of triacylated lipoproteins on the mycobacterium. TLR2/1 activation by *M. leprae* induces the production of TNF-α (as part of the acute inflammatory response), and of IL-12 (an important cytokine for the Th1 cell polarisation); thereby they participate in the defense against the pathogen [4]. Figure 1.

Some of the proteins of *M. leprae* can similarly activate TLR2; the major membrane protein II (MMP-II) is an example of this. It can stimulate the production of IL-12p70 in dendritic cells, though the inhibition of TLR2 in these cells through the use of anti-TLR2 antibodies demonstrates a clear IL-12p70 decrease after MMP-II stimulation [5].

The main TLR4 ligand is the lipopolysaccharide (LPS) of Gram-negative bacteria. *M. leprae* is able to activate this receptor, but thus far the ligands have not been identified [6]. A possible TLR4 activator could be the heat-shock protein 10 (HSP-10). *In vitro* studies in which macrophages are stimulated with the HSP-10 homologue protein of *Chlamydophila pneumoniae* show the production of cytokines TNF-α, IL-1β and IL-6.

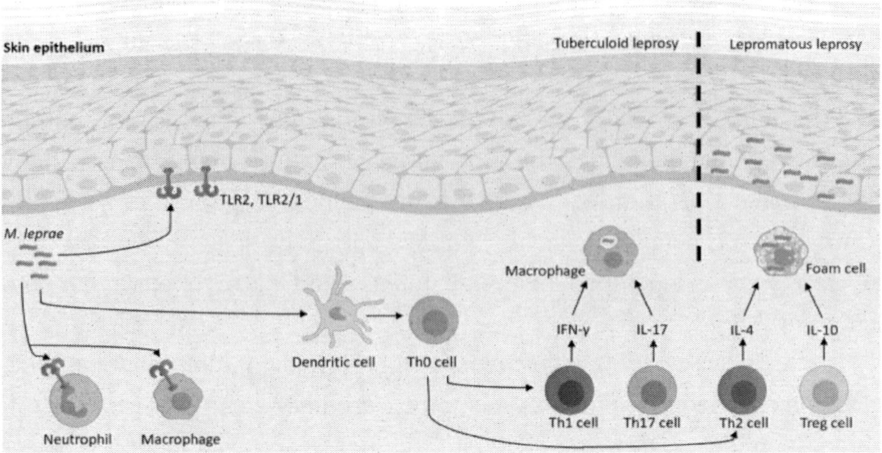

Figure 1. General aspects of the leprosy immune response. The immune response against M. leprae begins by the TLRs activation that are found in epithelial cells and innate immunity cells. The activation of these receptors induces the cytokine and chemokine production that will help in the activation and migration of other immune cells. Additionally, dendritic cells that are found in the skin will catch mycobacteria antigens, and then migrate to lymph nodes and present these antigens to Th0 cells (CD4+ T naïve cells), which will be polarized in 2 main subpopulations depending on the type of leprosy. In patients with tuberculoid leprosy, the T cells will differentiate into Th1 cells, productors of IFN-γ, and together with Th17 cells, they will increase the microbicide activity of macrophages, and in this way, they will eliminate M. leprae. In patients with lepromatous leprosy, Th0 cells will differentiate into Th2 cells, which together with Treg cells, they contribute to the bacillus survival (Created with BioRender.com).

When TLR4 in macrophages is blocked by anti-TLR4 antibodies and then stimulated with HSP-10, a clear reduction in these cytokines' production is observed [7]. Until now, there is only one study reported in which HSP-10 of *M. leprae* has been utilised. The authors proved *in vitro* that this protein increases the proliferation of peripheral blood mononuclear cells [8].

TLRs expression can be mediated by certain cytokines. Th1 cytokines (principally IFN-γ) increase TLR1 expression in monocytes and dendritic cells; however, IL-4 diminishes TLR2 expression. Tuberculoid leprosy patients present an increased expression of TLR1 and TLR2 in the lesions, while lepromatous leprosy patients have a decreased expression of these TLRs. This can be explained through the cytokine profile, since it directs the immune response to one or the other pole of the disease, with tuberculoid leprosy patients and lepromatous leprosy patients showing high levels of IFN-γ and IL-4, respectively [4, 6].

TLR expression and function in different cells can be affected by genetic factors such as mutations or epigenetic modifications in promoter sequences and the presence of single nucleotide polymorphisms (SNPs). SNPs can provoke changes in the gene expression and the structure of the encoded protein; this is a consequence of possible amino acid changes in the sequence, therefore causing defects in the encoded receptor's function [9].

The rs4833095 SNP in the *TLR1* gene exchanges a cytosine for a thymine, and it is associated with an increase in the susceptibility to leprosy in a Brazilian population carrying the T allele. In this study, the rs3804099 SNP in the *TLR2* gene is associated with an increase in IL-17 production in carriers of the T allele [10].

Innate Immunity Cells

Neutrophils are the most abundant leukocytes in mammals. These cells can eliminate pathogens through a variety of effector mechanisms: phagocytosis, reactive oxygen species (ROS) production, microbicidal protein degranulation activity, and neutrophil extracellular traps (NETs) liberation [11].

M. leprae activates neutrophils in the many subclassifications of the disease, and these cells do not differ in their microbicidal abilities. When they are activated, neutrophils increase their motility, even though it has been proved that neutrophils from lepromatous leprosy patients have motility deficiencies. However, it is unknown if these neutrophils are capable of mycobacterial elimination, since leprosy patients have neutrophils loaded with *M. leprae* in the peripheral blood. Nevertheless, neutrophils have a significant role in erythema nodosum leprosum (ENL), due to their possible contribution to the symptoms present in this leprosy reaction (this will be discussed later) [12].

Macrophages are the phagocytic cells par excellence and differentiate mainly into two different populations: M1 and M2. M1, or classically activated macrophages, are stimulated by IFN-γ, TLR ligands and some bacterial compounds such as LPS.

They are characterised by an increase in their microbicidal abilities (ROS and reactive nitrogen species production) and cytokine production (TNF-α, IL-6, IL-12, IL-23); additionally, M1 macrophages actively participate in the Th1 immune response. M2 macrophages are polarised by IL-4 and IL-13 cytokines; they participate primarily in tissue remodelling and produce large quantities of anti-inflammatory cytokines (IL-10 and TGF-β) [13].

In leprosy, macrophages have a key role in the disease pathology. The first *in vitro* studies of these cells revealed interesting information. Macrophages obtained from lepromatous leprosy patients' blood were unable to eliminate *M. leprae*, whereas macrophages from tuberculoid leprosy patients eliminated this mycobacterium [14].

In 1963, Rudolf Virchow described certain changes in the macrophage morphology in the leprosy patients' lesions. The macrophages in lepromatous leprosy lesions have a foamy appearance due to the large number of bacilli inside them. Macrophages in the lesions of tuberculoid leprosy are believed to be active and are similar to epithelial cells; because of this, they are named epithelioid or Virchow cells [4].

Depending on the type of leprosy, there are differences in the macrophage phenotype. In paucibacillary leprosy lesions and in the beginning of the reverse reaction (RR, a type of leprosy reaction), M1 macrophages predominate, whereas in multibacillary leprosy lesions, M2 macrophages with an anti-inflammatory profile are present. Also, M2 macrophages present in lepromatous leprosy lesions have an increase in iron storage (which is characteristic of M1 macrophages); this increases the iron deposits in macrophages and contributes to the *M. leprae* proliferation [15]. Figure 2.

Dendritic cells (DCs) are the most specialised antigen-presenting cells. They are responsible for trapping incoming pathogens, carrying them to lymph nodes and presenting the antigens to naïve T lymphocytes.

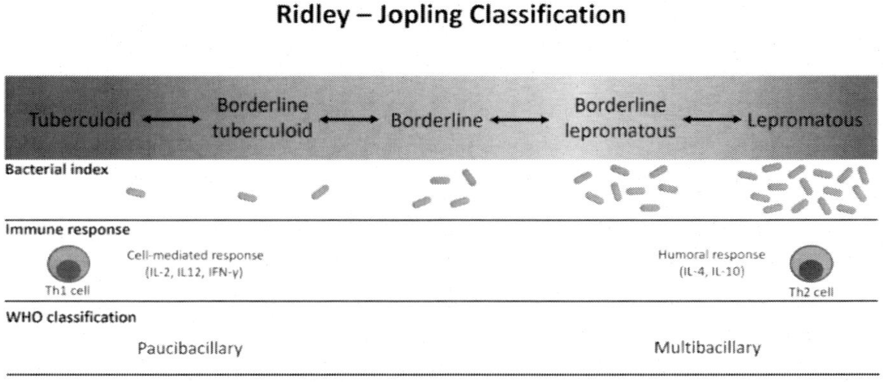

Figure 2. General aspects of the leprosy disease. According to Ripley-Jording, patients with leprosy can be classified in a 5-group spectrum. The poles, tuberculoid leprosy (TL) and lepromatous leprosy (LL), and between them there are 3 groups under the Borderline denomination. If the disease characteristics are closer to the tuberculoid pole, it is denominated Borderline tuberculoid (BT); and if it is closer to the lepromatous pole, it is called Borderline lepromatous (BL). Borderline-Borderline (BB) is when it has characteristics from both poles. Patients with TL show an immune response mediated by Th1 cells. And patients with LL show an immune response mediated by Th2. Finally, the WHO classifies leprosy patients in just two groups: paucibacillary and multibacillary (Created with BioRender.com).

There are two main dendritic cell populations, differing principally in their phenotypic properties and functions: plasmacytoid DCs and classical or conventional DCs. Plasmacytoid DCs are important for viral immunity due to their ability to produce type I interferons in response to viral infection. Classical DCs have as a primary function the stimulation of T lymphocytes, and which subdivide according to their localisation, function and phenotype done. In humans, a classical DC that we find in skin is the Langerhans cell in the epidermis. In the dermis, we find $CD14^+$ DCs (involved in humoural immunity) along with $CD1a^+$ DCs [16].

CD1 are a glycoprotein family with a structure similar to the major histocompatibility complex (MHC). They have the ability to join with lipidic antigens, and in this way DCs can present them to a particular type of CD1-specific T lymphocyte and contribute to the defense against a microorganism whose cell wall is mainly composed of glycolipids (i.e., mycobacterium). In leprosy, CD1 expression on DCs varies in the skin depending on the leprosy type. In tuberculoid leprosy lesions, DCs express more CD1 than in lepromatous leprosy lesions, so the expression of this glycoprotein could have an important role in the immunity against microbial pathogens [17].

Finally, in lepromatous leprosy, deficiencies in DC maturation have been reported. This is mainly attributed to the fact that *M. leprae* contains phenolic glycolipid I (PGL-1), a virulence factor with the ability to alter DC maturation; it also alters the DC's ability to present antigens, and in this way, PGL-1 allows the survival of the mycobacterium [18].

Adaptive Immunity

The adaptive immune system is characterised by its specificity and immunological memory. There are two classes of adaptive memory: the humoural immunity, in which antibodies and B lymphocytes participate in the defense; and cellular immunity, represented by T lymphocytes ($CD4^+$ and $CD8^+$). In order for the adaptive immune response to function properly, in addition to the TCR-MHC (T lymphocyte/antigen presenting cell) interaction, the participation of co-stimulatory molecules is necessary. Co-stimulatory molecules are important to ensure optimal activation of T lymphocytes. The interaction between B7-1/2 (CD80/CD86) and ICAM-1 molecules present in cells presenting antigens to their coreceptors LFA-1 and CD28 in T lymphocytes has a vital role in the signal transduction and in T lymphocytes adhesion. In borderline lepromatous leprosy/lepromatous leprosy patients, a decrease in CD28 and B7-1 expression has been reported; this could be responsible for the alteration in the B7-1/CD28 signalling pathway caused by *M. leprae* antigens in T lymphocytes [19].

Whereas tuberculoid leprosy patients present an adequate T lymphocyte response and undetectable antibody levels, patients with lepromatous leprosy show high levels of antibodies and a poor cell-mediated immune response. This correlates with the lepromin skin test, which is positive in tuberculoid leprosy patients (due to a good cellular response) and negative in lepromatous leprosy patients (due to the characteristic anergy of this disease pole) [20].

Adaptive Immunity Cells

The $CD4^+$ T or T helper lymphocyte (Th) differentiation is a key process in the generation of the adaptive immune response. After the T cell receptor (TCR) activation, naïve Th cells are polarised into distinct subtypes, the most common of which are Th1, Th2, Th17 and Tregs cells. These subpopulations of Th cells differ according to the transcription factor they will express, the cytokines that can induce them and the cytokines they will produce. Many factors are involved in the newly activated naïve T lymphocyte polarisation towards Th1 and Th2 effector T lymphocytes. Some of these factors are: the cytokine microenvironment, the pathway and dose of antigen administration, the type of antigen-presenting cell that stimulates the T lymphocyte, and the signal intensity of the T cell receptor upon joining the MHC. However, the incorrect polarisation of Th cells could lead to autoimmune diseases and chronic infectious diseases [21, 22].

The response of polarised T cells (Th1/Th2) against *M. leprae* is a critical element in the leprosy pathogenesis, as well as in variations in the clinical manifestations. The tuberculoid type of the disease is characterised by a Th1 immune response; these cells are polarised by IL-12 (an important cytokine in Th1 cell differentiation) and IFN-γ stimulation [23]. Figure 1.

IFN-γ is the main cytokine of Th1 cells, as well as NK cells and $CD8^+$ T cells done. The functions of this cytokine include the activation of the antigen presentation process during T cell priming, the increase in the MHC II expression and the DCs maturation. In macrophages, IFN-γ increases phagocytic ability, NO and ROS production and M1 polarisation. Patients with tuberculoid leprosy have few well-defined skin lesions, with little (or no) presence of bacilli in them. This is because tuberculoid leprosy patients present a cell-mediated immunity with a Th1 cytokine profile, which is very effective against intracellular bacteria [23].

The lepromatous pole of the disease is characterised by a Th2 cell-mediated immune response. These cells produce primarily IL-4, IL-10, and TGF-β, cytokines that antagonise Th1 cells and inactivate the microbicidal activity of macrophages, thereby contributing to the proliferation of *M. leprae* [24]. Figure 1.

Although leprosy presents mostly an adaptive immune response of type Th1 or Th2, it has also been suggested that other Th cell subpopulations could be implicated in the disease pathogenesis, as in the case of Th17 and Tregs cells.

Th17 cells function in elimination of bacteria and fungi. They are induced by IL-6 and TGF-β cytokines, and they produce the proinflammatory cytokines IL-17A, IL-17F and IL-22, which are involved in the production of antimicrobial peptides, tissue repair and remodelling, and neutrophilia. Also, Th17 cells mediate their function through neutrophil recruitment, macrophage activation and improvement in the Th1 cell response. In leprosy, Th17 cells have been found in *borderline* cases, while in the tuberculoid classification of the disease, an increase in the expression of IL-17 has been found. Therefore, Th17 cells could have a role in the modulation of macrophage activity, since IL-17 induces TNF-α, IL-6, and iNOS production, leading to reactive oxygen species production, and helping to eliminate the bacillus [21, 24].

Tregs cells have immunosuppressor activity. There are two main subtypes: $CD4^+CD25^+$ Tregs and inducible Tregs, both with the ability to suppress Th1 and Th17 cell functions. In addition to this, Tregs suppress other cells by their IL-10 and TGF-β production, and in dendritic cells, Tregs inhibit IL-12 and MHC II expression. In leprosy, Tregs cells could have an important part in the lepromatous pole of the disease, since it has been proven that there is an increase in this T lymphocyte subpopulation. In this way, Tregs could contribute to the characteristic anergy of this pole due to the inhibition of the Th1 immune response. Therefore, they could contribute to the proliferation of this bacillus [21].

The *borderline* conditions of this disease are immunologically dynamic.

As they approach the lepromatous pole, there is a decrease in the cell-mediated immunity with an increase in the bacillar load and a higher number of lesions; the opposite occurs when they approach the tuberculoid pole [25].

Leprosy Reactions Immunology

The leprosy reactions are acute inflammatory episodes that occur along the chronic evolution of the disease. These reactions present an intense neural inflammation, which could result in permanent loss of motor and sensory functions. They are classified into two main types: the type I reaction, also known as reverse reaction (RR), and the type II reaction, also known as erythema nodosum leprosum (ENL) [25].

The type I reactions can occur before, during or after treatment (although they are more frequent after treatment). They are present in the dimorphic types of the disease (*borderline*), and they are due to a transitory increase in the cell-mediated immunity (upgrading reaction) against *M. leprae* antigens. This produces a phenomenon of hypersensitivity that manifests itself at the cutaneous level with an increase in the inflammation of pre-existent lesions and in nerve damage, leaving irreversible sequelae. There is an improvement of the immunity with a worsening of the clinical manifestations. This could be due to the significant increase in the innate immune response during the RR, as well as to the increase in the Th1 lymphocyte population, which results in the increase of proinflammatory cytokines IL-1, IL-2, IL-6, IL-8, IFN-γ and TNF-α, thus contributing to the inflammatory process of the RR [25, 26].

Also, in type I reactions there is a decrease in the cellular immunity (downgrading reaction), which is present in borderline (BB) and borderline lepromatous (BL) patients. These cases evolve to the lepromatous pole due to the decrease in the immune response, allowing an increase in the proliferation of mycobacteria, and therefore an increase in the bacteriological index of the patients [26]. Figure 2.

The type II reactions occur due to an immunological complication and are present in the BL and lepromatous leprosy (LL) types. These reactions are characterised by painful subcutaneous erythematous nodules that can ulcerate. ENL has been described as a condition mediated by immune complexes, and it is generally induced by the deposition of these complexes, generating vasculitis. In addition, there is a significant infiltration of neutrophils in the lesions, activation of the complement cascade and production of the IL-4, IL-5, IL-10, IL-6, IFN-γ and TNF-α cytokines. TNF-α is implicated in the pathogenesis of neural damage that is produced in leprosy [26].

Finally, during ENL, neutrophils could contribute to the characteristic symptoms of this leprosy reaction. This is because of the high expression of CD64 in neutrophils, a marker that is associated with an improvement in neutrophil function. Also, during ENL, patients show an increase in histone-DNA complexes and an increase in the apoptotic neutrophil proportion in comparison with BL/LL patients [12]. Figure 2.

Based on the above, it is likely that during ENL, the increase in histone-DNA complexes could come from NETosis neutrophils, and in this way, they could contribute to the symptoms that characterise this leprosy reaction. However, more studies are needed to prove the presence of NETs in patients with ENL.

REFERENCES

[1] Oktaria, S., Effendi, E. H., Indriatmi, W., van Hees, C. L., Thio, H. B., Sjamsoe-Daili, E. S. "Soil-transmitted Helminth Infections and Leprosy: A Cross-sectional Study of the Association between Two Major Neglected Tropical Diseases in Indonesia". *BMC Infectious Diseases,* 16 (2016). doi:10.1186/s12879-016-1593-0.

[2] Hart, B. E., Tapping, R. I. “Genetic diversity of Toll-like receptors and immunity to *M. leprae* infection”. *Journal of Tropical Medicine,* 1 (2012). doi: 10.1155/2012/415057.

[3] Krutzik, S. R., Tan, B., Li, H., Ochoa, M. T., Liu, P. T., Sharfstein, S. E., Graeber, T. G., Sieling, P. A., Liu, Y. J., Rea, T. H., Bloom, B. R., Modlin, R. L. "TLR Activation Triggers the Rapid Differentiation of Monocytes into Macrophages and Dendritic Cells". *Nature Medicine,* 11, (2005). doi:10.1038/nm1246.

[4] Modlin, R. L. "The Innate Immune Response in Leprosy". *Current Opinion in Immunology*, 22 (2010): 48 - 54. doi:10.1016/ j.coi.2009.12.001.

[5] Maeda, Y., Mukai, T., Spencer, J., Makino, M. "Identification of an Immunomodulating Agent from *Mycobacterium Leprae*". *Infection and Immunity*, 73 (2005). doi:10.1128/iai.73.7.4458.2005.

[6] Krutzik, S. R., Ochoa, M. T., Sieling, P. A., Uematsu, S., Ng, Y. W., Legaspi, A., Liu, P. T., Cole, S. T., Godowski, P. J., Maeda, Y., Sarno, E. N., Norgard, M. V., Brennan, P. J., Akira, S., Rea, T. H., Modlin, R. L. "Activation and regulation of Toll-like receptors 2 and 1 in human leprosy". *Nature Medicine*, 9 (2003). doi: 10.1038/nm864.

[7] Zhou, Z., Wu, Y., Chen, L., Liu, L., Chen, H., Li, Z., Chen, C. "Heat shock protein 10 of Chlamydophila pneumoniae induces proinflammatory cytokines through Toll-like receptor (TLR) 2 and TLR4 in human monocytes THP-1". *In Vitro Cellular and Developmental Biology – Animal*, 47 (2011). doi: 10.1007/s11626-011-9441-4.

[8] Chua-Intra, B., Peerapakorn, S., Davey, N., Jurcevic, S., Busson, M., Vordermeier, H. M., Pirayavaraporn, C., Ivanyi, J. "T-cell recognition of mycobacterial GroES peptides in Thai leprosy patients and contacts". *Infection and immunity*, 66 (1998).

[9] Vidya, M. K., Kumar, V. G., Sejian, V., Bagath, M., Krishnan, G., Bhatta, R. "Toll-like receptors: Significance, ligands, signaling pathways, and functions in mammals". *International Reviews of Immunology*, 37 (2018). doi: 10.1080/08830185.2017.1380200.

[10] Santana, N. L., Rêgo, J. L., Oliveira, J. M., Almeida, L., Braz, M., Machado, L. M., Machado, P. R., Castellucci, L. C. "Polymorphisms in Genes TLR1, 2 and 4 Are Associated with Differential Cytokine and Chemokine Serum Production in Patients with Leprosy". *Memórias Do Instituto Oswaldo Cruz*, 4 (2017). doi:10.1590/0074-02760160366.

[11] Pruchniak, M. P., Arazna, M., Demkow, U. "Life of Neutrophil: From Stem Cell to Neutrophil Extracellular Trap". *Respiratory Physiology and Neurobiology*, 1 (2013). doi: 10.1016/j.resp.2013.02.023.

[12] Schmitz, V., Tavares, I. F., Pignataro, P., Machado, A. M., Pacheco, F. D. S., Dos Santos, J. B., da Silva, C. O., Sarno, E. N. "Neutrophils in Leprosy". *Frontiers Immunology*, 10 (2019). doi: 10.3389/fimmu.2019.00495.

[13] Aras, S., Zaidi, M. R. "TAMeless Traitors: Macrophages in Cancer Progression and Metastasis". *British Journal of Cancer*, 11 (2017). doi:10.1038/bjc.2017.356.

[14] Birdi, T. J., Antia, N. H. "The macrophage in leprosy: a review on the current status". *International journal of leprosy and other mycobacterial diseases*, (1989).

[15] Pinheiro, R. O., Schmitz, V., Silva, B. J. A., Dias, A. A., de Souza, B. J., de Mattos Barbosa, M. G., de Almeida Esquenazi, D., Pessolani, M. C. V., Sarno, E. N. "Innate Immune Responses in Leprosy". *Frontiers in Immunology*, 9 (2018) doi:10.3389/fimmu.2018.00518.

[16] Ueno, H., Palucka, A. K., Banchereau, J. "The expanding family of dendritic cell subsets". *Nature Biotechnology*, 28 (2010). doi: 10.1038/nbt0810-813.

[17] Sieling, P. A., Jullien, D., Dahlem, M., Tedder, T. F., Rea, T. H., Modlin, R. L., Porcelli, S. A. "CD1 Expression by Dendritic Cells in Human Leprosy Lesions: Correlation with Effective Host Immunity". *The Journal of Immunology*, 162 (1999).

[18] Spencer, J. S., Brennan, P. J. "The role of Mycobacterium leprae phenolic glycolipid I (PGL-I) in serodiagnosis and in the pathogenesis of leprosy". *Leprosy review*, 82 (2011).

[19] Agrewala, J. N., Kumar, B., Vohra, H. "Potential role of B7-1 and CD28 molecules in immunosuppression in leprosy". *Clinical and Experimental Immunology,* 111 (1998). doi: 10.1046/j.1365-2249.1998.00463.x.

[20] Nath, I., Saini, C., Valluri, V. L. "Immunology of leprosy and diagnostic challenges". *Clinics in Dermatology*, 33. (2015) doi: 10.1016/j.clindermatol.2014.07.005.

[21] Sadhu, S., Mitra, D. K. "Emerging Concepts of Adaptive Immunity in Leprosy Front Immunol". *Frontiers in immunology*, 9 (2018) doi: 10.3389/fimmu.2018.00604.

[22] Fang, D., Zhu, J. "Dynamic balance between master transcription factors determines the fates and functions of CD4 T cell and innate lymphoid cell subsets". *The Journal of experimental medicine*, 7 (2017). doi:10.1084/jem.20170494.

[23] Lee, A. J., Ashkar, A. A. "The Dual Nature of Type I and Type II Interferons". *Frontiers in immunology*, 9 (2018). doi:10.3389/fimmu.2018.02061.

[24] de Sousa, J. R., Sotto, M. N., Simões Quaresma, J. A. "Leprosy As a Complex Infection: Breakdown of the Th1 and Th2 Immune Paradigm in the Immunopathogenesis of the Disease." *Frontiers in immunology*, 8 (2017). doi:10.3389/fimmu.2017.01635.

[25] Fonseca, A. B., Simon, M. D., Cazzaniga, R. A., de Moura, T. R., de Almeida, R., Duthie, M. S., de Jesus, A. R. "The influence of innate and adaptative immune responses on the differential clinical outcomes of leprosy". *Infectious diseases of poverty*, 6 (2017). doi:10.1186/s40249-016-0229-3.

[26] Naafs, B., van Hees, C. L. "Leprosy type 1 reaction (formerly reversal reaction)". *Clinics in Dermatology*, 34 (2016). doi: 10.1016/j.clindermatol.2015.10.006.

[27] Costa, P. D. S. S., Fraga, L. R., Kowalski, T. W., Daxbacher, E. L. R., Schuler-Faccini, L., Vianna, F. S. L. "Erythema Nodosum Leprosum: Update and challenges on the treatment of a neglected condition". *Acta Tropica*, 183 (2018). doi: 10.1016/ j.acta tropica.2018.02.026.

In: Leprosy: From Diagnosis to Treatment
ISBN: 978-1-53616-629-3
Editor: Daniel L. Knuth

Chapter 3

IMMUNOLOGICAL ASPECT OF LEPROSY

Nyoman Suryawati*

Dermatology and Venereology Department, Faculty of Medicine, Udayana University, Denpasar, Bali, Indonesia

ABSTRACT

Leprosy is an infectious skin disease caused by *Mycobacterium leprae* (*M. leprae*). *M. leprae* can invade keratinocytes cells, macrophages cells, dendritic cells (DCs), and Schwann cells. *M. leprae* can induce various clinical manifestation depending on genetic susceptibility and the host immune system. The host immune system plays a vital role in leprosy pathogenesis. Leprosy patients can present as a broad spectrum of clinical manifestation, which are classified as paucibacillary (PB) type and multibacillary (MB) type. In the course of the disease, leprosy patients can experience episodes of acute inflammatory reactions known as leprosy reactions. Leprosy reactions are complications that may occur before, during, or after treatment, and cause further neurological damage that can cause chronic disabilities. This review will discuss the role of the immune response in leprosy pathogenesis and leprosy reactions.

* Corresponding Author's E-mail: suryawati@unud.ac.id.

Keywords: innate immune, adaptive immune, leprosy pathogenesis, leprosy reaction

INTRODUCTION

Leprosy, also known as Hansen's disease, is a chronic infectious disease. It mainly affects the skin, the peripheral nerves, mucosal surfaces of the upper respiratory tract, and the eyes. Leprosy is known to occur at all ages ranging from early infancy to ancient age. It is curable, and immediate treatment averts most disabilities.

The World Health Organization (WHO) considers leprosy as a complex disease that has a significant impact on health, social, economic, and psychological problems (Castro, Erazo, and Gunturiz 2018). Leprosy is still a major public health problem, especially in many third world countries. Seventeen endemic countries accounted for 95% (215,938) of new cases in 2010, 55.5% (126,800) of them detected in India, followed by Brazil (15.3% -34,894), and Indonesia (7.5% – 17,260) (Schreuder, Noto, and Richardus 2016; Marciano et al. 2018). There is an upward trend in both leprosy prevalence and the detection of new leprosy cases. Leprosy prevalence in Brazil changed from 4.71/10,000 inhabitants in 2000 to 1.56/10,000 inhabitants in 2010. In 2016, the ratio 1.10/10,000 was considered medium (1.0 to 4.9/10,000 inhabitants) (Marciano et al. 2018). In Indonesia, the number of new cases detected between 2011 and 2012 appears to have slightly declined, with 20,023 cases in 2011 and 18,994 cases in 2012 (Rahman et al. 2018).

Leprosy was regarded as a stigmatized disease until today. It causes discrimination and stigmatization in patients. Related to the delayed case finding, diagnosis, and treatment, patients often experience isolation, rejection by society, family, and social network. It contributes to the transmission of the disease and disabilities of patients (Castro, Erazo, and Gunturiz 2018).

In 2016 the WHO launched the program to reinvigorate efforts for leprosy control and to avoid disabilities, especially among children affected by the disease in endemic countries. Worldwide, two to three million people are estimated to be permanently disabled because of leprosy. India has the most significant number of cases, with Brazil second, and Burma third. Although the reported number of registered cases worldwide has declined in the past two decades, the number of new cases registered each year has remained almost the same.

PATHOGENESIS

Leprosy is an infectious disease caused by *Mycobacterium leprae* (*M. leprae*), a rod-shape bacteria, acid-fast, 1.5-8 μm in length, and 0.2-0.5 μm in width (Graca, Nardi, and Paschoal 2014). This bacteria can last up to 36 hours at room temperature, and its multiplication in the host system takes 11-16 days. The survival of *M. leprae* in the host cells depends on the structure of the cell wall (Graca, Nardi, and Paschoal 2014). The bacteria cell wall contains proteins, phenolic glycolipids, arabinoglycan, peptidoglycan, and mycolic acid (Sasaki et al. 2001; Jin, Ahn, and An 2018). *M. leprae* prefers the colder areas of the human body (Jin, Ahn, and An 2018). It can invade keratinocytes cells, macrophages cells, dendritic cells (DCs), and Schwann cells (Graca, Nardi, and Paschoal 2014).

The exact transmission mechanism of leprosy is not known. The primary mode of transmission of *M. leprae* is direct and prolonged contact with untreated cases. However, 30 to 60% of new cases have not been in contact with people with leprosy, indicating the existence of an environmental source such as water and soil close to center with endemic leprosy (Castro, Erazo, and Gunturiz 2018).

Human infections usually happen in youth (mostly in infancy), when *M. leprae* is inhaled through the respiratory tract upon close contact with leprosy patients (Castro, Erazo, and Gunturiz 2018). After entering the body, bacilli migrate towards the neural tissue and enter the Schwann cells. Bacteria also in macrophages, muscle cells, and endothelial cells of blood vessels. It starts multiplying slowly (about 12-14 days) within the cells, gets liberated from the destroyed cells, and enter of the unaffected cells (Mawardi 2018).

After the bacilli multiplication, bacterial load increase in the body, the immunological system will recognize the infection. Lymphocytes and histiocytes (macrophages) invade the infected tissue. At this stage, the clinical manifestation may appear as the involvement of nerves with impairment of sensation and skin patch. If it is not diagnosed and treated in early stages, further progress of the diseases is dependent on the strength of the patient's immune response (Mawardi 2018).

Specific and effective cell-mediated immunity (CMI) protects a person against leprosy. When specific CMI is effective in eliminating the infection in the body, lesions heal spontaneously, or it produces a paucibacillary (PB) type of leprosy. If the CMI is deficient, the disease spreads uncontrolled and produces multibacillary (MB) type leprosy with multiple systems involved. Sometimes the immune response is abruptly altered, either following treatment or due to the improvement of immunological status, which results in the inflammation of skin or nerves or other tissues called a leprosy reaction (Wankhade et al. 2019).

Clinical Manifestation of Leprosy

M. leprae can induce various clinical manifestation depends on genetic susceptibility, and the host immune system (Castro, Erazo, and Gunturiz 2018). Due to its chronic and subclinical progression, leprosy often represents a diagnostic challenge and depends on a high degree of suspicion by the clinician. Even with proper antimycobacterial treatment, leprosy follows up remains challenging. The difficulties in diagnosing and managing leprosy are particularly evident in the transplant setting, where leprosy is not initially suspected, and the diagnosis is only revealed through the histopathology examination of cutaneous lesions (Vieira et al. 2017).

Leprosy is diagnosed by finding at least one of the following cardinal signs such as definite loss of sensation in a pale (hypopigmented) or reddish skin patch; thickened or enlarged peripheral nerve, with loss of sensation and/or weakness of the muscle supplied by that nerve; presence of acid-fast bacilli in a slit-skin smear (Weltgesundheitsorganisation 2012).

In 1981, the WHO Study Group on Chemotherapy of Leprosy for Control Programmes classified leprosy as paucibacillary (PB) and multibacillary (MB), according to the degree of skin-smear positivity (Weltgesundheitsorganisation 2012; Fonseca et al. 2017). PB patients are characterized as having less than five skin lesions and rare bacilli, while the lesions in multibacillary patients are disseminated with voluminous bacilli (Schmitz et al. 2019). PB included indeterminate (I), polar tuberculoid (TT), and borderline tuberculoid (BT) cases in the Ridley-Jopling classification, with a bacterial index of <2 at all sites in the initial skin smears. MB included polar lepromatous (LL), borderline lepromatous (BL) and mid-borderline (BB) cases in the Ridley-Jopling classification, with a bacterial index of >2+ or more in the initial slit skin-smears (Weltgesundheitsorganisation 2012; Fonseca et al. 2017).

INDETERMINATE (I)

Indeterminate is the initial stage of leprosy, which served as the first sign of the disease in about 20-80% of the patients, often in the examination of family contacts of an index case (Kumar, Uprety, and Dogra, n.d.; Fischer 2017). It is generally believed that CMI response against M. leprae is not well developed in this early presentation (Kumar, Uprety, and Dogra, n.d.) This condition is hard to diagnose, even with the other tests such as histopathology, bacteriology, or molecular biology test (Fischer 2017).

The skin lesion is characterized by hypopigmented macules, hypochromic, with no erythema or infiltration, which can be found anywhere on the skin body (Fischer 2017). Sensory loss is unusual in this type. Initial signs can be found at the end of the disease stage, a subtle of neurological deficits such as decreased sweating and a loss of thermosensitivity. The pain sensitivity is still intact. These symptoms indicate the transition to the next advanced stage (Fischer 2017; Kumar, Uprety, and Dogra, n.d.).

The Polar Tuberculoid (TT)

Tuberculoid leprosy (TT) characterized by one or two larger macular hypopigmented or erythematous anesthetic lesions that have a sharp and often raised margin or appear as scaly plaques. The first type of lesion is a macule that has erythema or hypochloremic and has a dry, hairless surface and a sharp outer edge and sensory damage. Foci of well-developed epithelloid cells, with or without Langhans giant cells, are encompassed by a zone of dense lymphocyte infiltration. The granuloma, which extends up to the epidermis, is without a clear intervening area (Jin, Ahn, and An 2018). Neural involvement in TT is uncommon and usually occurs as a result of the extension of the infection through the superficial cutaneous branch. Due to the high CMI in TT patients, the lesions may heal on their own in the majority of the patients (Kumar, Uprety, and Dogra, n.d.).

Borderline Tuberculoid (BT)

In Borderline Tuberculoid (BT), the macules or plaques resemble TT leprosy in appearance and sensory loss.BT type characterized by a smaller average size, are more numerous, the surface is less dry, the outer edges are less defined, hair growth is less affected, and thickening of the nerves. The cytology and composition of the granuloma are typically indistinguishable from those of TT. The most distinguishing characteristic is the presence of a clear subepidermal zone; however, it is very narrow.

The granulomas can be distinguished from BB based on epithelial cell focalization near the peripheral lymphocyte region or occasionally by the presence of Langhans giant cells. The nerve bundles within the granuloma are generally grossly swollen and infiltrated, and innervation is greatly diminishing (Jin, Ahn, and An 2018). In BT patients, there is an asymmetrically and irregularly thickened of the nerves. The patient may present with anesthesia and motor deficits. The nerves are severely involved in episodes of reaction in BT patients (Kumar, Uprety, and Dogra, n.d.).

BORDERLINE BORDERLINE (BB)

In cases of Borderline Borderline (BB), the lesion size and the number is between that of TT and LL, moderate anesthesia and exhibits a typical 'punched-out' or 'hole-in-cheese' appearance. The essential defining characteristic is the presence of epithelial cells diffused throughout the granuloma and not by the lymphocyte zone. The epithelial cells are well-developed but generally not as large as those in TT leprosy. BB lesions contain no Langhans giant cells, and lymphocytes are present, they are highly diffuse. Besides, the nerve bundles exhibit moderate Schwann cell proliferation, but they are usually recognizable without much difficulty (Jin, Ahn, and An 2018).

BB is the most immunologically unstable portion of the borderline spectrum. The nerve involvement is variable in BB. If downgrading from BT, there may be asymmetrical nerve thickening, but if upgrading from BL, the nerve thickening may be more symmetrical. Nerve involvement may be severe in the case of type 1 reactions (Kumar, Uprety, and Dogra, n.d.).

BORDERLINE LEPROMATOUS (BL)

Borderline Lepromatous (BL) lesions tend to be numerous and particularly macular and consist of lacerations, papules, and nodules. There are two types of BL leprosy: (1) granulomas that include histiocytic cells that cannot be classified as epithelial cells but tend to evolve into epithelial cells and (2) the M. leprae host cells that consist of histiocytes that are typical to exhibit foamy changes; however, they do not produce large globes. The granulomas can be distinguished from LL granulomas by the presence of dense lymphocytic infiltration (Jin, Ahn, and An 2018). In BL, the peripheral nerve trunks are thickened and tend to be symmetrical. The nerve damage is not as severe as in BT, and the corresponding anesthesia and paresis are usually not seen in the early stages of the disease. Symmetrical anesthesia involving hand and feet are seen in the course of the disease (Kumar, Uprety, and Dogra, n.d.).

LEPROMATOUS LEPROSY (LL)

Lepromatous Leprosy (LL) lesions typically consist of erythematous macules, papules, and nodules, which are widespread and can occasionally become diffuse without defined lesions. Also, the lesions may appear similar to TT but with more BT and BL characteristics. Sensory and motor loss usually occurs in the nerves near TT lesions but may be more prevalent in BL and LL leprosy. Nerve damage is a common form of sensory loss and occurs at the final stages of LL leprosy. The ulnar and median (clawed hands), the common peroneal (foot drop), the posterior tibial (claw toes and plantar insensitivity) and the facial, radial cutaneous and great auricular nerves are involved. Occasionally, progressive multibacillary LL leprosy can result in the loss of the eyebrows and eyelashes, nasal septal perforation with a collapsed nose and hoarseness (Jacobson and Krahenbuhl 1999).

Moreover, the granuloma is composed of histiocytes that exhibit a varying degree of fatty changes, characterized by the production of foam cells and globi. In LL type we can find numerous globi or massive foamy changes. Lymphocytes are usually deficient and diffuse if they are present. Nerves can show structural damage but do not exhibit cell penetration or cuffing (Jin, Ahn, and An 2018).

The impairment of CMI in LL patients makes the uncontrolled multiplication and dissemination of leprae bacilli. LL can appear de novo (polar lepromatous leprosy/LLp) due to the highly anergic state of the individual or may downgrade from the BT or BL spectrum in the absence of treatment (subpolar lepromatous leprosy/LLs) (Kumar, Uprety, and Dogra, n.d.).

THE ROLE OF GENETIC IN LEPROSY

Several studies have demonstrated genetic predisposition in leprosy, with the most common associated with alleles of genes that encode human leucocyte antigens (HLA), located on chromosome 6q21. Case-control studies have shown an association of HLA gene regions with susceptibility or resistance to leprosy in different populations, such as HLADRB1 in Chinese communities; HLA-DR2 (DRB1 * 16) and HLA-DQ alleles in India, Thailand, and Brazil (Graca et al., 2014). In leprosy, genome-wide association study (GWAS) and replication studies provided insights into disease pathogenesis and revealed an unexpected overlap in the genetic control of leprosy and its clinical presentations with common inflammatory disorders such as Crohn's disease (Dallmann-Sauer, Correa-Macedo, and Schurr 2018).

IMMUNE RESPONSE IN LEPROSY

For the immunologists, however, leprosy still garners much attention mainly because *M. leprae* infection which evokes distinct polarized T cell responses in humans, which correlates with the clinical manifestations. In the post-elimination era, renewed interest in leprosy has developed owing to the reemergence of infection. Newer insights into the mode of transmission, pathogenesis, as well as newer diagnostic techniques with the use of microsatellite typing of mycobacterial strains, has been obtained. However, it continues to be a particularly devastating disease, especially in the developing and the underdeveloped world, due to the deformities and morbidities associated with it, and one of the most critical factors contributing to it are leprosy reactions (Wankhade et al. 2019).

Polarization of the immune response specific to M. leprae is an essential element in the pathogenesis of leprosy and in determining the clinical manifestation (Fonseca et al. 2017; D. Montoya and Modlin 2010). In leprosy skin lesion $CD4^+$ T cell predominates in tuberculoid leprosy (T-lep form), whereas $CD8^+T$ cell predominates in lepromatous leprosy (L-lep form). The $CD4^+$ T cells produce the type-1 or Th1 cytokine pattern including interferon-gamma (IFN-ɣ) predominate in T-lep lesions, whereas $CD8^+T$ cells produce the type-2 or Th2 cytokine pattern including interleukin (IL)-4 predominate in L-lep lesion (D. Montoya and Modlin 2010; Fonseca et al. 2017).

The immune response of TT patients is characterized by Th1 cytokines such as IFN-ɣ, IL-2, IL-15, and tumor necrosis factor (TNF), vigorous T cell response to M. leprae antigens, and containment of the bacilli in the well-formed granuloma. In TT patients, activated macrophages that resemble epithelial cells, and $CD4^+$ T cell is predominant cell type (Fonseca et al. 2017).

A Th2 immune profile characterizes the immune response in LL patients with the production of IL-4, and IL-10, and activation of T regulatory (T reg), robust but not protective antibody production including the formation of immune complexes. Lesion of LL patients relative deficient in $CD4^+$ T cells has numerous $CD8^+$ T cells, and macrophages heavily infected with bacilli that develop a characteristic foamy appearance (Fonseca et al. 2017).

The borderline forms are immunologically dynamic. There is a progressive reduction of the T cell-mediated response from the BT to the BB and BL forms, accompanied by more numerous neurocutaneous lesions and an increase of bacterial load (D. M. Scollard et al. 2006).

The pathogenesis of nerve destruction varies accordingly, the clinical form of the disease (Pinheiro et al. 2018). *M leprae* activates TLR 2 dan TLR1 in Schwann cells, which leads explicitly to TT leprosy. Although the cell-mediated immune response is most active in TT leprosy, it can also activate the apoptosis gene and consequently cause nerve damage in cases of TT leprosy (Jin, Ahn, and An 2018). In the pure neural leprosy (PNL), bacilli are rarely detected despite clinical neurological impairment. In MB cases showed macrophages in considerable numbers within the nerve, bacilli are more significant in number often as large bundles or globi (Pinheiro et al. 2018).

INNATE IMMUNE RESPONSE IN LEPROSY

M. leprae transmitted from infected to a healthy person through aerosol containing bacteria. The most common route is likely to be the upper airways, indicating that interaction between *M. leprae* and the human host begins in the nasal mucosa (Klatser 1993; PatrocÃ-nio et al. 2005; Araujo et al. 2016; Pinheiro et al. 2018). The protective mucosal innate mechanism in the respiratory tract may contribute to the low infectivity of *M. leprae* after the exposition. The viable bacilli have been found for at least two days in discharge nasal secretion (Pinheiro et al. 2018).

The cell that mediated the innate response-able to recognize, phagocytose, and destroy the foreign invader. The cell of the innate immune system is equipped with germline-encoded pattern recognition receptors (PRRs), which recognize pathogen-associated molecular patterns (PAMPs) (Modlin 2010). *M. leprae* bacteria initially recognized by several innate immune receptors, including toll-like receptors (TLRs). *M. leprae* predominantly activates TLR2/1 heterodimer express in macrophages in the skin, which mediates cell activation to kill the bacteria (Fonseca et al. 2017; D. Montoya and Modlin 2010).

PRRs that detect PAMPs mediate the first line of the interaction between M. leprae and the host. These recognition receptors are expressed primarily by phagocytic cells such as macrophages and DCs. Previous studies have demonstrated the versatility of these receptors and the signaling cascades that can develop. Many theories have proposed for the immune mechanism in leprosy, which based on the course of the response involving the relationship between TLRs, DCs, macrophages, and lymphocytes. Among the receptors expressed by phagocytic cells, TLR2 and TLR4 are the two significant receptors involved in the development of the immune response by recognition of the *M. leprae* PAMPs (de Sousa, Sotto, and Simões Quaresma 2017).

The ability of TLRs to trigger a direct antimicrobial activity is central to their role in innate immunity. The induction of the antimicrobial peptide required the presence of 25D-sufficient human serum. There is some evidence that indicates that vitamin D antimicrobial pathway may contribute to disease outcome in leprosy (D. Montoya and Modlin 2010).

Macrophage Cell

In Metchikoff's model of innate immunity, phagocytosis will continue after the recognition of microbial pathogens. A vital cell of the mammalian innate immune system that mediates phagocytosis of the microbial pathogen is the Mϕ macrophage (D. Montoya and Modlin 2010). Macrophages are the cell population that plays a pivotal role in the interaction between the bacillus and host (de Sousa, Sotto, and Simões Quaresma 2017; Moraes, Silva, and Pinheiro, n.d.).

In addition to their phagocytic function, Mϕ also mediates an antimicrobial activity against infectious agents (D. Montoya and Modlin 2010; de Sousa, Sotto, and Simões Quaresma 2017). Mϕ infiltration is prominent in all lesions, Mϕs in the self-healing T-lep form are well-differentiated and rarely contain bacteria. Mϕs in the disseminated L-lep form characterized by abundant intracellular bacilli and foam cell formation as the result of the accumulation of host- and pathogen lipids (D. Montoya and Modlin 2010).

During infection, *M. leprae* invades DCs and macrophages mediated by pathogen recognition through TLR, inducing the expression of activation signals and directing a cascade of immunological events. The *M. leprae* antigen exposure drives the enhancement of proinflammatory cytokines such as TNF-α, and IFN-γ produced by neutrophils and lymphocytes, and stimulates the synthesis of nitric oxide (NO), orchestrating an effective cell-mediated immune response (Carvalho et al. 2018). In leprosy, both TNF-α and IFN-γ have been shown to bind to the cellular receptor of the macrophages, thereby changing the behavior of Mϕ macrophages, which undergo phenotypic modification to become M1 inflammatory macrophages. M1 macrophages produce inflammatory cytokines and enzymes such as induced nitric oxide synthase (iNOS), which influences the production of NO and consequently generates free radicals that destroy the bacillus (de Sousa, Sotto, and Simões Quaresma 2017).

An alternative pathway has identified in the lepromatous form, which is activated owing to the presence of M2 macrophages that produce anti-inflammatory cytokines (IL-4, IL-10, and IL-13), growth factors [transforming growth factor (TGF)-β and basic fibroblast growth factor (bFGF)], and enzymes such as arginase 1 and enzyme indoleamine 2, 3-dioxygenase (IDO) that contribute to the development of immune-suppressive mechanisms as well tissue repair. Therefore, the response of M2 macrophages plays a vital role in the immunopathology of the lepromatous form of the disease, because these cells express the scavenger receptor (CD163) that may contribute to entry into the bacillus cell (de Sousa, Sotto, and Simões Quaresma 2017).

Dendritic Cells (DCs)

The ability of the innate immune system to instruct the adaptive T cell response is a part of effective host defense against intracellular pathogens. The DCs mediate the instructive role of the innate immune system as antigen-presenting cells. The DCs process antigens and present them to $CD8^+$Tcell via class I MHC molecules and to the $CD4^+$ T cell via class II MHC molecules (D. Montoya and Modlin 2010).

Some evidence indicates a role for DCs in the immune response to *M. leprae*. Concerning the DCs response, more recent studies have identified a variety of cell subtypes that modulate the initial construction of the immune response in the polar forms of the disease. In this context, the presence of the DCs of the epidermis ($CD1a^+$) and langerin ($CD207^+$) show particularly increased expression in the tuberculoid form (de Sousa, Sotto, and Simões Quaresma 2017). Concerning the inflammatory infiltrates, the immunostaining of dermal dendrocytes (FXIIIA$^+$) and plasmacytoid dendritic cells (CD123$^+$) predominantly detected near the vessels and granulomas in the tuberculoid form. These findings demonstrated that the presence of DCs in epidermis or areas close to the infiltrate participates in the development of an effective immune response against *M. leprae*.

KERATINOCYTE CELLS

Keratinocytes and the epidermis play an essential role in the innate immune response against M. leprae (Lyrio et al. 2015; Jin, Ahn, and An 2018). Keratinocytes express mannose-binding receptor (KCMR), TLRs, and Class II MHC antigen, which has identified as a source of cytokines, chemokines, and antimicrobial peptide (Jin, Ahn, and An 2018). Keratinocytes as a source of cytokines and chemokines that are critical for recruiting DCs, T cells, and neutrophils to the site of infection (Lyrio et al. 2015). Human keratinocytes have been shown to envelop and destroy M. leprae in vitro and subsequently exhibit changes in the expression of surface molecules and cathelicidin as well as secrete TNF-α and IL-1β (Lyrio et al. 2015; Jin, Ahn, and An 2018). There was a report of the invasion of keratinocytes and the secretion of cytokines and chemokines by immune cells, which suggests that keratinocytes play an essential role in the immune response to infection with M. leprae (Jin, Ahn, and An 2018).

ADAPTIVE IMMUNE RESPONSE IN LEPROSY

The host's immune system affects the clinical manifestation of leprosy. Strong cell-mediated immunity and low humoral immunity characterize the response to tuberculoid (TT) leprosy, whereas the opposite in LL leprosy (Jin, Ahn, and An 2018). In the tuberculoid form (T-lep), the bacilli are rare, and the immune response is characterized by a CD4$^+$T Cell infiltrate and IFN-γ transcriptional signature, resulting in effective microbial response in macrophages (D. J. Montoya et al. 2019). In the T-lep, the lesions are granulomatous, and the individual displays a strong cell-mediated immune response (T helper-1/Th1) that prevents the proliferation of the bacillus (Aarao et al. 2018).

In the lepromatous form (L-lep) is characterized by abundant bacilli, B cells, or plasma cells, and the expression of a type I IFN gene program that suppresses macrophage antimicrobial activity (D. J. Montoya et al. 2019). In L-lep, the cell-mediated immune response is characterized by an anti-inflammatory cytokine profile (Th2) that contributes to the multiplication of the bacillus in macrophage phagosomes. In the borderline form, the patients exhibit immunological and histopathological characteristics that vary between those of the tuberculoid and lepromatous types (Aarao et al. 2018).

The T and B lymphocytes play crucial roles in the immune response since they participate in mechanisms that lead to the development of the microbicidal or humoral response in the spectrum of the disease. The two main types of T lymphocytes that are a most extensive study in the $CD4^+$ T cell response pathway are the Th1 lymphocytes associated with the tuberculoid form and the Th2 lymphocytes associated with the lepromatous form. $CD8^+$ T cells are primarily involved in the development of cytotoxicity. Studies have shown that the $CD8^+$ T cells participate in mechanisms that lead to the destruction of the bacillus in coinfection with HIV in a reverse reaction. In this context, by recognizing virus-infected cells, $CD8^+$ T cells would promote the release of granzymes and perforins that destroy the coinfected cells in patients with a type-1 reverse reaction. The response of the B lymphocytes is primarily associated with the humoral response, and some studies on leprosy have demonstrated increased expression of CD20 in the tuberculoid form and borderline tuberculoid form in a reverse reaction (de Sousa, Sotto, and Simões Quaresma 2017).

Immune Response in Leprosy Reaction

Almost half of the leprosy patients develop reaction episodes, i.e., worsening of the previous lesions or appearance of new inflamed lesions and neuritis due to exacerbation of the immune response in the patient (Vieira et al. 2017). These flare-ups referred to as leprosy reactions (Fischer 2017). Clinically, the reaction described as the appearance of symptoms and signs of acute inflammation in lesions of a leprosy patient (Shah et al. 2019). It is generally a manifestation of a sudden impairment in the immunological balance established over the preceding disease course between the pathogen and the infected individual. These immune reactions can occur even after successful treatment (Fischer 2017).

Immunologically, reactions are episodes of acute hypersensitivity to bacterial antigens, due to a disturbance in the pre-existing immunological balance (Shah et al. 2019). One-third of people with leprosy develop pathologic immune reactions, either reversal reaction (RR) or erythema nodosum leprosum (ENL) (Vieira et al. 2017). Leprosy reactions, reversal reactions/RR, and erythema nodosum cause irreversible nerve damage, handicaps, and deformities (Fava et al. 2017). Leprosy reactions are directly associated with the morbidity of leprosy (Vieira et al. 2017).

Type I Leprosy Reaction (Reversal Reaction/RR)

Reversal reaction (RR) occurs in 30% of patients and involves a sudden activation of an inflammatory response to *M. leprae* antigens. RR reflects a switch from a Th2-predominant toward to Th1 response. (Fonseca et al. 2017). RR manifests clinically as an upgrade from the L-lep to the T-lep form of the disease, associated with a change from a type I to type II IFN response (D. J. Montoya et al. 2019). Both innate and adaptive immune responses involved in the RR pathogenesis. RR lesion is associated with type-IV or delayed-type hypersensitivity reaction (Fonseca et al. 2017).

Clinical symptoms may present with complaints of burning, stinging sensations in the skin lesions. Sign manifestations increase inflammation become erythematous swollen and may be tender, edema of extremities or face frequently accompanied by nerve involvement, rapid swelling with severe pain (neuritis), and sometimes loss of nerve function (Mawardi 2018).

TYPE II LEPROSY REACTION (ERYTHEMA NODOSUM LEPROSUM/ENL)

Type 2 leprosy reaction or erythema nodosum leprosum (ENL) is a type III immunological reaction (Vieira et al. 2017; Wankhade et al. 2019). ENL occurs most commonly in the lepromatous pole (BL, and LL), and can present before initiation, during or after completion of multidrug therapy (MDT) (Wankhade et al. 2019). Over 50% of lepromatous leprosy patients and 25% of borderline lepromatous leprosy patients experienced ENL before MDT. In this reaction, there is an exacerbated humoral immune response with an increased synthesis of IgG1 (Fava et al. 2017)(Fava et al. 2017).

ENL characterized by crops of transient, coppery tender nodules, and plaques with systemic symptoms of fever and malaise, and the involvement of other organ systems such as the eyes, testes, nerves, liver, and kidney (Vieira et al. 2017; Wankhade et al. 2019). ENL can manifest as mild and severe form. Severe ENL includes necrotic ENL or erythema nodosum necroticans (ENN), which is a rare presentation seen in around 8% of patients (Wankhade et al. 2019). Other uncommon and severe variants of ENL, such as ulceronecrotic, pustular lesions, vesiculobullous, Sweet's syndrome (SS)-like, erythema multiforme (EM)-like, Lucio phenomenon (LP), and reactive perforating type have reported in the literature (Suryawati and Saputra 2018; Wankhade et al. 2019). Due to their atypical morphology, these variants can mimic many other conditions. (Wankhade et al. 2019).

ENL is usually initiated by the deposition of immune complexes and activation of the complement cascade, resulting in vasculitis or a type -III hypersensitivity reaction (Fonseca et al. 2017). ENL is often described as a neutrophilic immune-complex-mediated condition, while there is evidence that T-cells further complicate the immunopathology. There were reports about the association between elevated levels of specific cytokines such as tumor necrosis factor (TNF)-α and other immunological factors with episodes of ENL (Polycarpou, Walker, and Lockwood 2017). Although ENL is considered a neutrophilic immune-complex mediated condition, there is a little information about the direct role of neutrophils in ENL and leprosy disease overall. Recent studies have shown a renewed interest in neutrophilic biology. One of the most existing recent discoveries was that the neutrophilic population is not homogeneous. Neutrophilic polarization leads to divergent phenotypes (e.g., a pro- and antitumor profile) that are dynamic subpopulations with distinct phenotypical and functional abilities. (Schmitz et al. 2019).

CONCLUSION

M. leprae can induce various clinical manifestation depends on genetic susceptibility and the host immune system. If leprosy is not diagnosed and treated in early stages, further progress of the diseases is dependent on the strength of the patient's immune response. Specific and effective CMI protects a person against leprosy. In the course of the disease, leprosy patients can experience episodes of acute inflammatory reactions called leprosy reactions. In a better immune system, lesions can heal spontaneously, or it produces a PB type of leprosy. Otherwise, the disease spreads uncontrolled and produces MB type leprosy with multiple system involved. The host's immune system plays a vital role in *M. leprae* pathogenesis, leprosy control, and avoiding disabilities.

REFERENCES

Aarao, TLS, JR de Sousa, ASC Falcao, LFM Falcao, and JAS Quaresma. 2018. "Nerve Growth Factor and Pathogenesis of Leprosy: Review and Update." *Frontiers in Immunology* 9: 1–8.

Araujo, Sergio, Larissa Oliveira Freitas, Luiz Ricardo Goulart, and Isabela Maria Bernardes Goulart. 2016. "Molecular Evidence for the Aerial Route of Infection of *Mycobacterium Leprae* and the Role of Asymptomatic Carriers in the Persistence of Leprosy." *Clinical Infectious Diseases* 63 (11): 1412–20. https://doi.org/10.1093/cid/ciw570.

Carvalho, Jairo Campos de, Marcelo Grossi Araújo, Jordana Grazziela Alves Coelho-dos-Reis, Vanessa Peruhype-Magalhães, Cláudio Caetano Alvares, Marcela de Lima Moreira, Andréa Teixeira-Carvalho, Olindo Assis Martins-Filho, and Márcio Sobreira Silva Araújo. 2018. "Phenotypic and Functional Features of Innate and Adaptive Immunity as Putative Biomarkers for Clinical Status and Leprosy Reactions." *Microbial Pathogenesis* 125 (December): 230–39. https://doi.org/10.1016/j.micpath.2018.09.011.

Castro, CM, L Erazo, and ML Gunturiz. 2018. "Strategies for Reducing Leprosy Stigma." *Mycobacterial Dis* 8: 1–4.

Dallmann-Sauer, Monica, Wilian Correa-Macedo, and Erwin Schurr. 2018. "Human Genetics of Mycobacterial Disease." *Mammalian Genome* 29 (7): 523–38. https://doi.org/10.1007/s00335-018-9765-4.

Fava, Vinicius M, Carolinne Sales-Marques, Alexandre Alcaïs, Milton O Moraes, and Erwin Schurr. 2017. "Age-Dependent Association of TNFSF15/TNFSF8 Variants and Leprosy Type 1 Reaction." *Frontiers in Immunology* 8 (February). https://doi.org/10.3389/fimmu.2017.00155.

Fischer, Marcellus. 2017. "Leprosy – an Overview of Clinical Features, Diagnosis, and Treatment." *JDDG: Journal Der Deutschen Dermatologischen Gesellschaft* 15 (8): 801–27. https://doi.org/10.1111/ddg.13301.

Fonseca, Adriana Barbosa de Lima, Marise do Vale Simon, Rodrigo Anselmo Cazzaniga, Tatiana Rodrigues de Moura, Roque Pacheco de Almeida, Malcolm S. Duthie, Steven G. Reed, and Amelia Ribeiro de Jesus. 2017. "The Influence of Innate and Adaptative Immune Responses on the Differential Clinical Outcomes of Leprosy." *Infectious Diseases of Poverty* 6 (1). https://doi.org/10.1186/s40249-016-0229-3.

Graca, CR, SMT Nardi, and DelArco Paschoal. 2014. "Update on Genetics of Leprosy." *Journal of Ancient Diseases & Preventive Remedies* 02 (01). https://doi.org/10.4172/2329-8731.1000109.

Jin, HS, KJ Ahn, and S An. 2018. "Importance of the Immune Response to Mycobacterium Leprae in the Skin." *Biomedical Dermatology* 2: 1–6.

Klatser, Paul R. 1993. "Detection of Mycobacterium Leprae Nasal Carriers in Populations for Which Leprosy Is Endemic." *J. Clin. Microbiol.* 31: 5.

Kumar, Bhushan, Shraddha Uprety, and Sunil Dogra. n.d. "Clinical Diagnosis of Leprosy." *Clinical Aspects*, 24.

Lyrio, Eloah CD, Ivy C Campos-Souza, Luiz CD Corrêa, Guilherme C Lechuga, Maurício Verícimo, Helena C Castro, Saulo C Bourguignon, et al. 2015. "Interaction of *Mycobacterium Leprae* with the HaCaT Human Keratinocyte Cell Line: New Frontiers in the Cellular Immunology of Leprosy." *Experimental Dermatology* 24 (7): 536–42. https://doi.org/10.1111/exd.12714.

Marciano, LHSC, AFF Belone, PS Rosa, NMB Caelho, CC Ghidella, SMT Nardi, WC Miranda, LV Barrozo, and JC Lastoria. 2018. "Epidemiological and Geographical Characterization of Leprosy in a Brazilian Hyperendemic Municipality." *Cad. Saúde Pública* 34: e00197216.

Mawardi, Prasetyadi. 2018. "Leprosy: The Ancient and Stubborn Disease." In *Current Topics in Tropical Emerging Diseases and Travel Medicine*, edited by Alfonso J. Rodriguez-Morales. IntechOpen. https://doi.org/10.5772/intechopen.79984.

Modlin, Robert L. 2010. "The Innate Immune Response in Leprosy." *Current Opinion in Immunology* 22 (1): 48–54. https://doi.org/10.1016/j.coi.2009.12.001.

Montoya, Dennis J, Priscila Andrade, Bruno JA Silva, Rosane MB Teles, Feiyang Ma, Bryan Bryson, Saheli Sadanand, et al. 2019. "Dual RNA-Seq of Human Leprosy Lesions Identifies Bacterial Determinants Linked to Host Immune Response." *Cell Reports* 26 (13): 3574-3585.e3. https://doi.org/10.1016/j.celrep.2019.02.109.

Montoya, Dennis, and Robert L. Modlin. 2010. "Learning from Leprosy." In *Advances in Immunology*, 105:1–24. Elsevier. https://doi.org/10.1016/S0065-2776(10)05001-7.

Moraes, MO, LRB Silva, and RO Pinheiro. n.d. "Innate Immunity." In *The International Textbook of Leprosy*, edited by DM Scollard and TP Gillis, 1–28. https://internationaltextbookofleprosy.org.

PatrocÃ-nio, Lucas Gomes, Isabela Maria Bernardes Goulart, Luiz Ricardo Goulart, JosÃ© AntÃ´nio PatrocÃ-nio, Frederico RogÃ©rio Ferreira, and Raul NegrÃ£o Fleury. 2005. "Detection of *Mycobacterium Leprae* in Nasal Mucosa Biopsies by the Polymerase Chain Reaction." *FEMS Immunology & Medical Microbiology* 44 (3): 311–16. https://doi.org/10.1016/j.femsim.2005.01.002.

Pinheiro, Roberta Olmo, Veronica Schmitz, Bruno Jorge de Andrade Silva, André Alves Dias, Beatriz Junqueira de Souza, Mayara Garcia de Mattos Barbosa, Danuza de Almeida Esquenazi, Maria Cristina Vidal Pessolani, and Euzenir Nunes Sarno. 2018. "Innate Immune Responses in Leprosy." *Frontiers in Immunology* 9 (March). https://doi.org/10.3389/fimmu.2018.00518.

Polycarpou, Anastasia, Stephen L. Walker, and Diana N. J. Lockwood. 2017. "A Systematic Review of Immunological Studies of Erythema Nodosum Leprosum." *Frontiers in Immunology* 8 (March). https://doi.org/10.3389/fimmu.2017.00233.

Rahman, EA, SV Muchtar, F Tabri, S Wahab, A Adriani, A Seweng, and R Sjahrir. 2018. "Evaluation of Interleukin-12 and Interleukin-4 Levels in Multibacillary-Type Leprosy Patient 12 Months After Rifampicin,

Ofloxacin, Minocycline Combination Therapy : A Randomised Study." *International Journal of Medical Reviews and Case Reports*.

Sasaki, Shin, Fumihiko Takeshita, Kenji Okuda, and Norihisa Ishii. 2001. "*Mycobacterium Leprae* and Leprosy: A Compendium." *Microbiology and Immunology* 45 (11): 729–36. https://doi.org/10.1111/j.1348-0421.2001.tb01308.x.

Schmitz, Veronica, Isabella Forasteiro Tavares, Patricia Pignataro, Alice de Miranda Machado, Fabiana dos Santos Pacheco, Jéssica Brandão dos Santos, Camila Oliveira da Silva, and Euzenir Nunes Sarno. 2019. "Neutrophils in Leprosy." *Frontiers in Immunology* 10 (March). https://doi.org/10.3389/fimmu.2019.00495.

Schreuder, Pieter AM, Salvatore Noto, and Jan Hendrik Richardus. 2016. "Epidemiologic Trends of Leprosy for the 21st Century." *Clinics in Dermatology* 34 (1): 24–31. https://doi.org/10.1016/j.clindermatol.2015.11.001.

Scollard, DM, LB Adams, TP Gillis, JL Krahenbuhl, RW Truman, and DL Williams. 2006. "The Continuing Challenges of Leprosy." *Clinical Microbiology Reviews* 19 (2): 338–81. https://doi.org/10.1128/CMR.19.2.338-381.2006.

Shah, Urvi H., Monal M. Jadwani, Sahana P. Raju, Pranav H. Ladani, and Neela V. Bhuptani. 2019. "Clinical and Histopathological Features in Lepra Reaction: A Study of 50 Cases." *International Journal of Research in Dermatology* 5 (2): 382. https://doi.org/10.18203/issn.2455-4529.IntJResDermatol20191766.

Sousa, Jorge Rodrigues de, Mirian Nacagami Sotto, and Juarez Antonio Simões Quaresma. 2017. "Leprosy As a Complex Infection: Breakdown of the Th1 and Th2 Immune Paradigm in the Immunopathogenesis of the Disease." *Frontiers in Immunology* 8 (November). https://doi.org/10.3389/fimmu.2017.01635.

Suryawati, Nyoman, and Herman Saputra. 2018. "Erythema Nodosum Leprosum Presenting as Sweet's Syndrome-like Reaction in a Borderline Lepromatous Leprosy Patient." *International Journal of Mycobacteriology* 7 (2): 191. https://doi.org/10.4103/ijmy.ijmy_49_18.Vieira, Ana Paula, Maria Angela Bianconcini Trindade, Flávio

Jota de Paula, Neusa Yurico Sakai-Valente, Alberto José da Silva Duarte, Francine Brambate Carvalhinho Lemos, and Gil Benard. 2017. "Severe Type 1 Upgrading Leprosy Reaction in a Renal Transplant Recipient: A Paradoxical Manifestation Associated with Deficiency of Antigen-Specific Regulatory T-Cells?" *BMC Infectious Diseases* 17 (1). https://doi.org/10.1186/s12879-017-2406-9.

Wankhade, VH, Pritica Debnath, RP Singh, Gitesh Sawatkar, and DM Bhat. 2019. "A Retrospective Study of the Severe and Uncommon Variants of Erythema Nodosum Leprosum at a Tertiary Health Center in Central India." *International Journal of Mycobacteriology* 8 (1): 29. https://doi.org/10.4103/ijmy.ijmy_174_18.

Weltgesundheitsorganisation, ed. 2012. *Eighth Report/WHO Expert Committee on Leprosy: Geneva, 12 - 19 October 2010*. WHO Technical Report Series 968. Geneva: World Health Organization.

In: Leprosy: From Diagnosis to Treatment ISBN: 978-1-53616-629-3
Editor: Daniel L. Knuth

Chapter 4

TREATMENT OF LEPROSY: CURRENT PRACTICE AND UPDATED WHO GUIDELINES

T. Pugazhenthan*[1], *MD and V. Sajitha*[2], *MBBS
[1]Pharmacology, All India Institute of Medical Sciences (AIIMS), Raipur, India
[2]Clinical, Central Leprosy Teaching and Research Institute (CLTRI), Chengalpattu, India

ABSTRACT

The treatment of leprosy is always based on the final clinical and laboratory confirmation of the diagnosis. The diagnosed patient must be treated for 6 months in case of paucibacillary and 12 months in case of multibacillary Further, precaution should be always taken to treat a confirmed disease than by trial or error method, as many diseases mimic leprosy. At present three drugs, Rifampicin, Dapsone and clofazimine are given ~~for~~ to multibacillary leprosy cases and two drugs, Rifampicin and Dapsone are given to paucibacillary leprosy cases. Both the cases are given drugs in Blister Calendar Packs (BCP). Recently, the World Health Organisation (WHO) has updated the guideline for the treatment of leprosy. The WHO has emphasized to use three drugs for 6 months and 12 months for the two types of leprosy paucibacillary and multibacillary, respectively. There is also a standard guideline to use certain regimen in case of individual drug relapse. In addition, chemoprophylaxis of contacts of confirmed leprosy cases have also been updated in the guideline. Besides the established drug regimine, there are also many alternate regimines followed in special cases of contraindication and due to adverse effects.In addition to the regular treatment regimine, the treatment of leprosy includes management of lepra reactions with Non Steroidal anti-Inflammatory Drugs (NSAIDS), steroids in needed cases, and clofazimine and thalidomide in special situation like erythema nodosum leprosum(ENL). Moreover, lots of immunosuppressants have also been tried in lepra reactions. All the aspects of the treatment will be detailed out throughout the chapters.

Keywords: Leprosy, Treatment, Single dose rifampicin, WHO, updated

INTRODUCTION

The treatment of stigmatised leprosy case has been standardized worldwide after the success of various clinical trials and based on which, WHO has issued recommendations issued in 1982 for successful implementation. The treatment of leprosy involves the combination of drugs termed as Multi-Drug Therapy (MDT) and the drugs include sulpha drug Dapsone, bacteriocidal drug rifampicin, and antiinflamamtory and bacteriostatic drug clofazimine. The WHO recommends combinational drugs, due to the resistance occurred because of the usage of monotheraphy dapsone [1].

NOTES ON INDIVIDUAL DRUGS [1, 2]

Rifampicin

Rifampicin is from gram-positive bacteria found in soil namely Amycolatopsis rifamycinica and it has been manufactured for usage since 1965 as well as it was initially synthesized in Italy. The core mechanism of the drug is that it causes the inhibition of bacterial RNA polymerase. Since it is acting at the genetic level, it has maximum bactericidal effect on the infectious mycobacterium species including tuberculosis bacilli. Since it is active on the replicating bacilli, dormant bacilli escape from its cidal action and that may lead to the current resistance rate of 5% in the relapsed leprosy cases. It is also a factor for combinational theraphy importance. Even though it is assumed to be the safest drug in pregnancy and in all age groups, it has severe side effects like hepatotoxicity of intrahepatic cholestasis nature.

Flu like symptom is common in rifampicin usage person, due to the hypersensitivity reaction stoppage in a few. Gastrointestinal symptoms like nausea, vomiting, diarrhea but it subsides in most of the patients where as rarely causes have to be taken care. The main troublesome complaint, that will be notified by the patients, is red-orange discoloration of body fluids (saliva,tears,urine). This should be properly counselled before dispensing the drugs.

In the treatment of all types of leprosy, the dose for adults is 600mg supervised once a month and a reduced dose is for children. The Patient is advised to consume drug with the food or little before.

Dapsone

The first used drug as monotherapy in the treatment of leprosy in 1941 was Dapsone that was manufactured in Germany long back in 1908 with the chemical structure of 4,4′- diaminodiphenylsulfone.The mechanism of action of the drug is by inhibiting bacterial folic acid synthesis by the competition with Para amino benzoate (PABA) for the active site of enzyme dihydropteroate synthatase and it has the function of bacteriostatic effect in regular dosage.

Dapsone is known for its side effects. It includes gastrointestinal symptoms, generalised fatigue and headache which are dose-dependent and due to its oxidative stress on the red cells, it causes hemolysis and formation of methemoglobin. It is in the case of glucose-6-phosphate dehydrogenase deficiency, the haemoglobin related complications are more. Due to the sulpha nature rare side effects like phototoxic reactions, urticarial is seen.

Fixed Drug Eruption (FDE), erythema multiforme, agranulocytosis, Drug Rash or reaction with Eosinophilia and Systemic Symptoms (DRESS) syndrome, and dapsone induce cholestatic hepatitis. The daily dose is 100mg in all forms of leprosy in adult and it should be reduced accordingly as per the weight in case of children.

Clofazimine

Clofazimine is a red dye which was synthesized in 1954. Next to Dapsone in Dublin, it was first used in Nigeria for the treatment of leprosy in 1959.

The important property of the drug is that apart from minor bacteriocidal effect, it also has good anti-inflammatory properties that are beneficial for multibacillary leprosy where there is a need of management of bacilli and the inflammation, due to massive destruction of bacilli. Because of these properties, it is suitable for treating type 2 leprosy reactions.

But this anti-inflammatory action is a delayed process and it will take around 6 weeks to develop. It is also seen that more than 75% of multibacillary leprosy patients treated will develop hyperpigmentation of the existing leprosy lesions.

This property of skin changes may resolve only after the treatment has been discontinued and very slowly over months and years, that is seen in young adults but rare in elderly people. This is troublesome in case of young female who are fair. It needs revision of regimine by early stoppage of clofazimine and that may sometimes lead to relapse and the occurrence of leprosy of pseudo-obstruction and abdominal pain reactions. Another feature of its usage in children is that it is given twice in a week for fear and weight reductions.

Treatment Regimens [2]

Two treatment regimens have been established by the WHO based on the field clinical findings as well as laboratory presence of leprae bacilli and they have been classified into PauciBacillary (PB) and MultiBacillary form (MB).

As per the existing guideline before the updated version, they differ with respect to multi drug combinations as well as total treatment duration (Table 1, Figure 1, Figure 2).

Table 1. Classification and Dosage of multidrug theraphy before updation

Age group	Dosage and frequency	Classification	Duration (Months)
Children <10 years old or < 40 kg	Rifampicin (10mg/kg) once month Clofazimine (6mg/kg) once a month and (1mg/kg) daily Dapsone(2mg/kg) daily	Multibacillary (MB)	12
	Rifampicin (10mg/kg) once month Dapsone(2mg/kg) daily	Paucibacillary (PB)	6
Children (10–14 years)	Rifampicin 450mg once a month Clofazimine 150mg once a month, 50mg daily Dapsone 50mg daily	Multibacillary (MB)	12
	Rifampicin 450mg once a month Dapsone 50mg daily	Paucibacillary (PB)	6
Adult	Rifampicin 600mg once a month Clofazimine 300mg once a month and 50mg daily, Dapsone 100mg daily	Multibacillary (MB)	12
	Rifampicin 600mg once a month Dapsone 100mg daily	Paucibacillary (PB)	6

Both the regimens have been administered as blister calendar pack and supplied on an outpatient (OPD) basis.

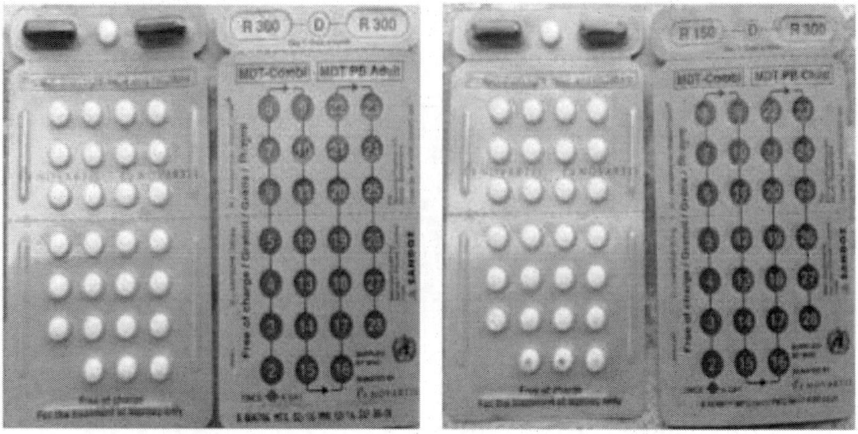

Paucibacillary (PB-A) Paucibacillary (PB-C)

Figure 1. The images of Paucibacillary regimine.

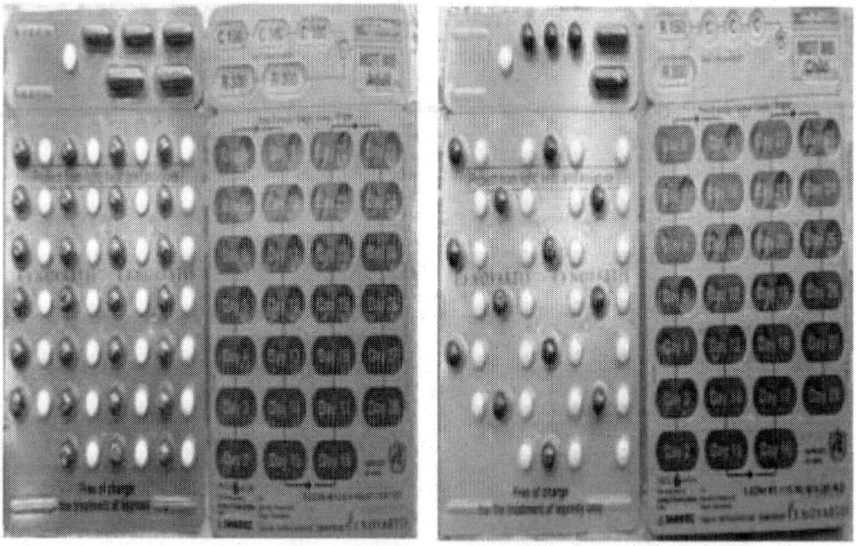

Multibacillary (MB-A) Multibacillary (MB-C)

Figure 2. The images of Multibacillary regimine.

Table 2. Classification and Dosage of multidrug therapy after recent updation

Age group	Dosage and frequency	Classification	Duration (Months)
Children <10 years old or < 40 kg	Rifampicin (10 mg/kg) once month Clofazimine (6 mg/kg) once a month and (1 mg/kg) daily Dapsone (2mg/kg) daily	Multibacillary (MB)	12
		Paucibacillary (PB)	6
Children (10–14 years)	Rifampicin 450 mg once a month Clofazimine 150 mg once a month, 50 mg daily Dapsone 50 mg daily	Multibacillary (MB)	12
		Paucibacillary (PB)	6
Adult	Rifampicin 600 mg once a month Clofazimine 300 mg once a month and 50 mg Daily Dapsone 100 mg daily	Multibacillary (MB)	12
		Paucibacillary (PB)	6

UPDATED GUIDELINE BY WHO [3]

Recently, World Health Organization (WHO) has updated treatment guidelines. Instead of the current regimens of two drugs, rifampicin and Dapsone in the treatment of Paucibacillary, it has now been advised to use 3 drugs with additional clofazimine for 6 months. This is based on various clinical studies that have shown promising improvement in both the clinical and histopathological disease status changes and to follow the existing treatment regimen in case of multibacillary (MB) leprosy for a period of 12 months that has to be completed within 18 months.

The dosage of the above mentioned three drugs for various adult population, especially the specified categories grouping of children under (10 - 14 years) and below < 10 years old or < 40kgs, remains the same as that of the existing scenario (Table 2).

Alternatives

Apart from those above mentioned two standard therapies, other class of drugs is used in special cases and they are fluroquilones group ofloxacin, tetracycline group minocycline and macrolides clarithromycin.

Efficacy

After four weeks of ofloxacin treatment with a dosage of 400mg QD, it is found that more than 99% of leprae bacilli have been killed. Minocycline given at a daily dose of 100mg shows a similar bactericidal profile with respect to killing of bacilli with the potency less than that of rifampicin. With regard to clarithromycin, four weeks of treatment with a dose of 500mg QD results in similar to 99% of killing of leprae bacilli.

Special Conditions

In Case of non Suitable to Use Dapsone

In Paucibacillary form, dapsone is substituted with clofazimine, as Rifampicin 600mg with clofazimine 50mg once a month followed by clofazimine 50mg daily for 28 days. Treatment period is same as 6 months and that has to be completed within nine months.

In the case of Multibacillary form, dapsone is replaced with either oflaxacin or minocycline.

So the drug rifampicin 450mg is given along with clofazimine 300mg, minocycline 100mg or ofloxacin 400mg once a month and this is followed by clofazimine 50mg and ofloxacin 400mg or minocycline 100mg OD, the treatment period remains the same with a total of twelve monthly doses and that has to be completed within 18 months.

In Case of Non Suitable to Use Rifampicin

In Paucibacillary leprosy, Dapsone 100mg and ofloxacin 400mg or minocycline 100mg once a month are followed by dapsone 100mg and ofloxacin 400mg or minocycline 100mg OD. The treatment period is 6 months and that has to be completed within nine months.

In Multibacillary leprosy, Dapsone 100mg and ofloxacin 400mg or minocycline 100mg with clofazimine 300mg once a month is followed by dapsone 100mg, ofloxacin 400mg or minocycline 100mg with clofazimine 50mg OD. Here, the treatment is to be completed after a total of 24 months but within 36 months.

In Case of Non Suitable to Use Rifampicin and Dapsone

In Paucibacillary leprosy, clofazimine 50mg and ofloxfacin 400mg or minocycline 100mg once a month followed by clofazimine and ofloxacin 400mg or minocycline 100mg OD are given for a treatment period of six months.

In case of Multibacillary leprosy, clofazimine 300mg with ofloxacin 400 mg, and minocycline 100mg once a month (for the first six months) with clofazimine 50mg, ofloxacin 400mg and minocycline 100mg OD. It is followed subsequently for another 18 months with clofazimine 300mg and ofloxacin 400mg or minocycline 100mg once a month followed by daily dose of clofazimine 50mg and ofloxacin 400mg or minocycline 100mg OD.

Here also, the total treatment has to be concluded after a total of 24 months doses within specified 36 months.

In Case of Non Suitable To Use Clofazimine

For, patients with multibacillary leprosy, the clofazimine is totally replaced and rifampicin 600mg, dapsone100mg, and ofloxacin 400mg or minocycline 100mg once a month is taken followed by dapsone 100mg and ofloxacin 400mg or minocycline 100mg OD for a duration of 12 months as well as it is to be completed within 18 months.

Regarding ROM (Rifampicin, Oflaxacin and Minocycline), treatment regimen is rarely used in high endemic set up countries.

TREATMENT OF LEPROSY REACTIONS

Lepra reaction is an important less bothered anticipated component and complication of leprosy requires treatment. It is the immunological response by the host immune system against the bacterial or drug components or antigen [4]. It should be managed rationally, as it is more important than managing the disease itself. Irrational management widely seen for lepra reaction leads to relapse of reaction symptoms. More frequently, it leads to reaction progression causing disability, if mismanagement of neuritis happens and above all, mostly the psychological stress that leads to sick and bad life.

Based on a recent web based survey, the knowledge of healthcare professionals mainly doctors in the management of classified lepra reaction is found to be very deficient [5].

There is also irrational management of reaction with currently available drugs.

TYPE 1 REACTION [6]

- Diagnosed Leprosy Case
- Paucibacillary (TT/BT)
- skin lesions suddenly become reddish, swollen, warm, painful/ tender but the rest of the skin is normal/fresh lesions
- General Condition is Good With Few Constitutional Symptoms (Fever)

Mild Type 1 Reaction

Symptoms

- Occurs in some of the pre-existing skin lesions only (Figure 3)
- Erythema and swelling of skin lesions without ulceration
- Nerves are not affected
- No constitutional symptoms
- No edema of hands and feet

Treatment

- Reassurance
- Continue multi drug therapy (MDT) if patient is on
- Aspirin 600mg 4th hourly (6 times a day)/ paracetamol 1 gram adult dose 4 times a day
- Tablet ranitidine 150 mg 1 BD till on aspirin
- Multivitamins, if possible

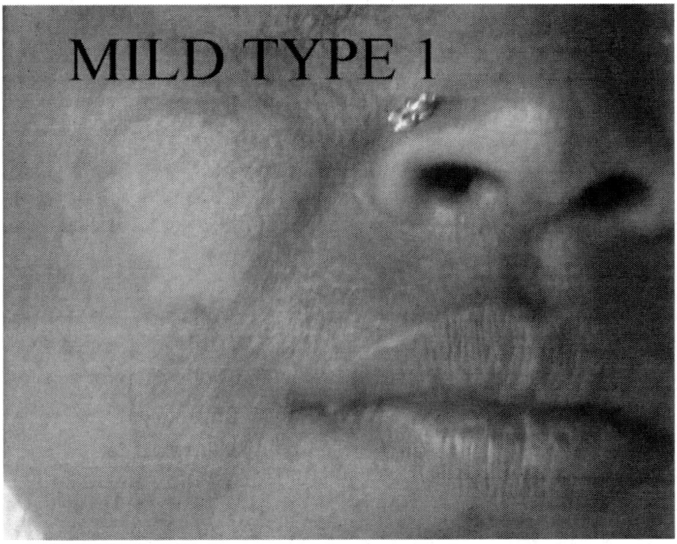

Figure 3. Reaction of pre existing lesion.

Severe Type 1 Reaction

Symptoms

- Red, painful, inflamed skin lesions with ulceration
- Pain or tenderness in one or more nerves with or without loss of nerve function
- An erythematous, swollen skin patch on the face around the eye
- Skin lesion overlying major nerve trunk
- Constitutional symptoms
- Marked oedema of the hands, feet or face (Figure 4)
- Clinically mild reaction not responding to NSAIDS for a period of 2 – 4 weeks.
- Increased or new muscle weakness noticed
- (motor loss)

Treatment

- Bed rest

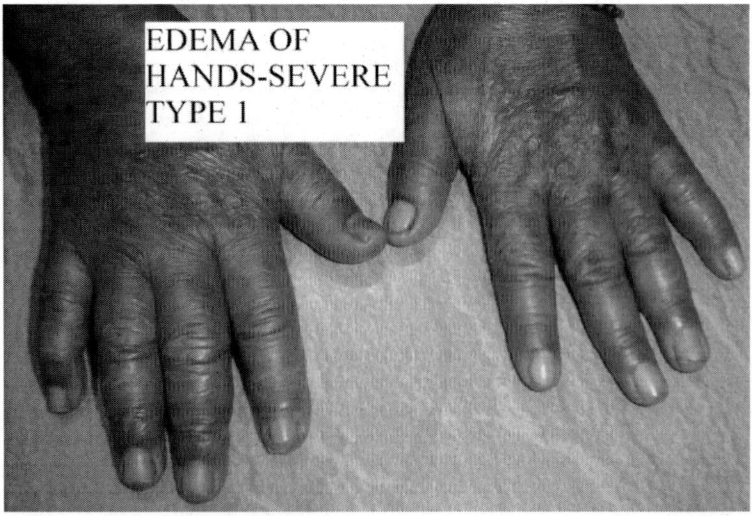

Figure 4. Edema and reaction of the hand.

- Rest to the affected nerve using splint
- Continue Multi Drug Therapy (MDT) if patient is on,
- Aspirin 600mg 4th hourly (6 times a day)/Paracetamol 1 gram adult dose 4 times a day
- Tablet ranitidine 150mg 1 BD till on aspirin
- Start tablet prednisolone (dose at 1mg/kg body wt/day) and it is given as a single morning dose after breakfast (consider giving tab ranitidine 150mg along with prednisolone).
- (Ii) After the reaction/inflammation is controlled, prednisolone is tapered by 10mg, fortnightly till the dose of 20mg/day.
- (Iii) Thereafter, prednisolone is tapered by 5mg/day, fortnightly till withdrawal.
- In case of neuritis, (inflammation of peripheral nerve trunk) the period of
- treatment is prolonged according to the response. From 20mg onwards (in table below), duration of each dose is increased for four weeks.
- Tablet calcium 1od
- Tablet alprax 0.25 to 0.5mg

TYPE II OR ERYTHEMA NODOSUM LEPROSUM (ENL)

- Diagnosed Leprosy Case
- Multibacillary (BB, BL, LL)
- Red, Painful, Tender, Cutaneous/Subcutaneous Nodules Appear (Not associated With Leprosy Patches).
- Appear Commonly on Face, Extensor Surfaces of Arms and Legs.
- General Condition is Poor with Prominent Fever and Malaise

Mild Type II Reaction Symptoms

- Intermittent crops of few ENL (Figure 5)
- Nerves are not affected
- Mild fever (less than 100 degree F) may or may not be present
- No other organs involved

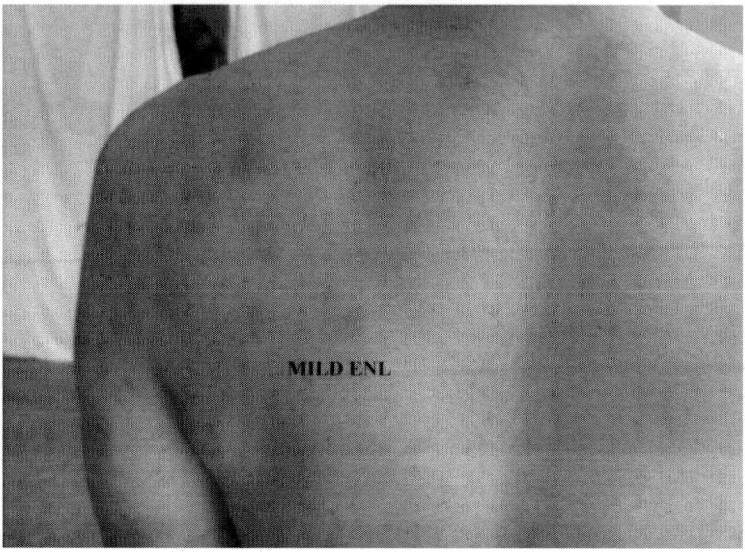

Figure 5. Crops of multiple nodules over the Back.

Treatment

- Reassurance
- Continue Multi Drug therapy (MDT) if patient is on, aspirin 600mg 4th hourly (6 times a day)/paracetamol 1 gram adult dose 4 times a day
- Tablet ranitidine 150mg 1 BD till on aspirin multivitamins, if possible

Moderate to Severe Type 2 ENL

Symptoms

- Red, painful, multiple/innumerable ENL in crops
- Pain or tenderness in one or more nerves with or without loss of nerve function
- ENL that becomes ulcerated (ENL necroticans) (Figure 6)
- Accompanied by a high fever (> 100 degree F)
- Pain and/or redness of the eyes with or without loss of visual acuity (involvement of eye)
- Generalized symptoms with painful swelling of the small joints with fever
- Recurrent ENL (more than four episodes in a year)
- Clinically mild reaction not responding to NSAIDS and/or within 2 – 4 weeksS.
- Enlargement of lymph glands/testes with pain or tenderness
- Involvement of other vital organs like kidneys, liver,
- Bone marrow, endocardium, etc.

Treatment

- Bed rest
- Rest to the affected nerve using splint
- Continue Multi Drug Therapy (MDT) if patient is on,
- Aspirin 600mg 4th hourly (6 times a day)/Paracetamol 1 gram adult dose 4 times a day
- Tablet ranitidine 150mg 1 BD till on aspirin
- Start tablet prednisolone (dose at 1mg/kg body wt/day) and it is given as a single morning dose after breakfast (consider giving tab ranitidine 150mg along with prednisolone).
- After the reaction/inflammation is controlled, prednisolone is tapered by 10mg, fortnightly till the dose of 20mg/day.

- Thereafter, prednisolone is tapered by 5 mg/day, fortnightly till withdrawal.
- In case of neuritis, (inflammation of peripheral nerve trunk) the period of treatment is prolonged according to the response. From 20mg onwards (in table below), the duration of each dose is increased to four weeks.
- Tablet calcium 1od
- Tablet alprax 0.25 to 0.5mg

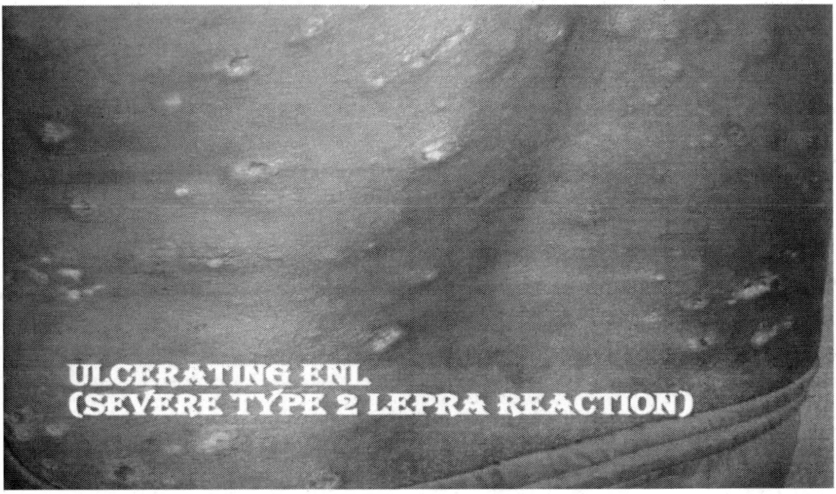

Figure 6. Multiple ulcerrated nodules at the back showing severity.

Steroid Dependent

✓ Clofazimine is given with corticosteroids in every case. one capsule (100mg) 3 times a day x 4 or more weeks (depending on the response) and then one capsule (100mg) 2 times a day x next 4 – 12 weeks, followed by One capsule (100mg) once a day x next 4 – 12 weeks or more

Steroid Contraindicated or Well Established Side Effects Need Steroids Stoppage

- ✓ Clofazimine plus
- ✓ Thalidomide
- Adult: 100 - 300mg once daily at bedtime. Reduce gradually by 50mg every 2 - 4 week, once a satisfactory response is achieved.
- Not for monotherapy, if moderate or severe neuritis is present. Max: 400mg/day.
- Patients < 50kg: initially, 100mg daily.

POINTS ON STEROIDS

1. Mild reaction – never/ever steroids
2. Absolute indication – severe reaction (neuritis)
3. Relative indication- to suppress severe inflammation in severe reaction(without neuritis)
4. Dose for absolute indication- 40mg/day or maximum up to 1mg/kg body weight
5. Dose for relative indication:
   - low initial dose(< 20mg/day) and upward titration (non critical situation)
   - high initial dose(> 30mg/day) and downward titration (critical situation)
6. Time of steroid intake – Preferably around 8.00 A.M (not interference in circadian rhythm and disturbance in sleep). Never split the required dose.
7. Frequency of steroid:
   - Oral Prednisolone - once a day (24hrs)
   - Injectable Dexametasone - alternative days (48hrs)
8. Dexametasone equivalences: 1mg of Dexametasone = 6.67mg of Prednisolone

- 2ml vial contains 8mg of Dexametasone
- So roughly 2ml is equal to 50mg of Prednisolone.

Chemoprophylaxis [7]

In a strategy to reduce the transmission of ongoing leprosy bacilli infection in the endemic area and other area of impotance, it has been decided by the World Health Organisation (WHO) to strongly implement chemoprophylaxis by bactericidal drug rifampicin for the close contacts of patients being diagnosed with confirmed leprosy in the current updated guideline [1]. It is based on an important COLEP2 randomized controlled trial and as an overview of the trial explained, it has shown that around 18869 (86.9%) of the 21711 defined contacts have been followed-up for 4 years. Among placebo group, around 91 out of 9452 contacts and in rifampicin group, around 59 out of 9417 have developed clinically confirmed leprosy.

It has also been found that in the intial first two years of treatment, there has been maximum 57% risk of reduction of developing any clinical leprosy. But, the result between placebo and rifampicin groups does not differ between two to four years.

From this, it has been concluded that SDR in leprosy contacts is associated with more than 50% (exactly 57%) reduction in the risk of developing clinical leprosy after two years and around 30% after a theoretical incubation period of around six years [8]. The findings provide evidence to use SDR as a cost effective, feasibile and more practical secondary preventive intervention approach for the close contacts of confirmed patients with all integrated leprosy control national programmes. In India, it has already been implemented with effect from 2nd October 2018.

CONCLUSION

Because of free availability of good drugs with best compliance, the prevalence rate has achieved a drastic decline. Since there are some proposals for uniform multi drug theraphy, early diagnosis with early treatment helps in the prevention of stigmatised disease in the society and also its complication.

Chemoprophylaxis and immunoprophylaxis defininetly will help in the prevention of transmission in the community.

REFERENCES

[1] Fischer, M. 2017. " Leprosy - an overview of clinical features, diagnosis, and treatment". *J. Dtsch. Dermatol. Ges.*, 15:801 - 27.

[2] Treatment of Leprosy. 2019. "WHO model prescribing information: Drugs used in Leprosy". Accessed June 7. http://apps.who.int/medicinedocs/pdf/h2988e/h2988e.pdf.

[3] National leprosy eradication program. 2019. "WHO guidelines 2018 for the Diagnosis, Treatment and Prevention of Leprosy". Accessed June 7. http://nlep.nic.in/pdf/WHO%20Guidelines%20for%20leprosy.pdf.

[4] *Treatment of lepra reactions.* 2019. Accessed June 7. http://apps.who.int / medicinedocs /en /d/Jh2988e/6.html# Jh2988e.6.

[5] Thangaraju, P., Venkatesan, S., Selvan, T. T., Sivshanmugam, E. et al. 2018. " The resurgence of leprosy in India:Findings from a survey assessing medical professionals' knowledge and preparedness". *Educations in the Health Professionals,* 1:24 - 7.

[6] Thangaraju, P. 2018. "First mobile application - Lepra reaction basic management guide - Stress on steroids". *Indian Journal of Drugs in Dermatology,* 4:85 - 6.

[7] Thangaraju, P., Venkatesan, S. 2019. "Single-dose rifampicin: What current World Health Organization guidelines emphasis and practical

special attention" ? *Hamdan Medical Journal,* Accessed June 7. DOI: 10.4103/HMJ.HMJ_4_19.

[8] Moet, F. Johannes, Pahan David, Oskam Linda, Richardus Jan H. 2008. "Effectiveness of single dose rifampicin in preventing leprosy in close contacts of patients with newly diagnosed leprosy: cluster randomised controlled trial" *British Medical Journal,* 336:761.

BIOGRAPHICAL SKETCH

T. Pugazhenthan

Affiliation: All India Institute of Medical Sciences, AIIMS, Raipur, India

Education: MBBS, MD, DNB, MNAMS, PGD.DIAB

Research and Professional Experience: My research area over the past few years were in the area of communicable tropical disease, leprosy in various aspects pertaining to various pharmacological interventions, basic pharmacology, and clinical Diabetology.

A. Leprosy:

- My research areas in leprosy include clinical aspects of leprosy, adverse effects of drugs used in leprosy, evaluating the efficacy of currently used anti-Lepra reaction drugs.
- One of the best contributions to the leprosy was the drug sensitivity analysis, which helped in framing the rational drug to be used in the central leprosy setting of our institute to prevent the resistance.

- Secondly, additional information on rifampicin mainly its nature of causing hyper pigmentation have been worked out and disseminated to the scientific community.
- Rational use of antibiotic is my core in leprosy too
- Drug utilization study and analysis of various sources of drugs information for rational prescription is the area of interest for me.
- Drug information deficiency in the drug sources available in india pertaining to thalidomoide, steroids and clofazimine.
- Single dose rifampicin integration in LCDC
- Vaccine mycobacterium indicus pranii integration in LCDC

B. Pharmacology:

- An important contribution which added to the management of diabetic micro vascular complication is the study done in basic pharmacology unit in PGIMER. It was targeting the renin Angiotensin system with combinational dose in diabetic nephropathy and retinopathy. As it was well established in the literature that targeting the RAS helps in diabetic nephropathy. Our study also confirmed the fact with additional information obtained in diabetic retinopathy that it also helps in preventing the early neuronal damage in diabetic eye.
- A positive response by antidepressant drug imipramine in the management of orofacial pain in tooth extracted patient was also found through a project.
- I have contributed in the molecular biology field in projects regarding the resistance pattern in enterobacteriace and helps in the control of resistance in future by adhering to the basic essential method by the doctors and health workers cleanness and hygiene.
- I have developed an mobile application for the teaching purpose in the steroid rationale usage

- Actively involved in the reporting of Adverse drug reaction and create awareness all the medical professionals in perusing the same.

C. Diabetology:

- An observational study regarding diabetes and HbA1c and diabetic keto acidosis has been evaluated which helps in assessing the doctors knowledge in these areas and steps were taken to enhance the knowledge in those management.

Professional Appointments:

Name of Organisation	Department & Postion Held	Durations
Postgraduate Institute of Medical Education and Research (PGIMER) Chandigarh	Pharmacology/ Junior Resident	2010-2013
Central Leprosy Teaching Research Institute (CLTRI), Chengalpattu	Clinical (Pharmacology)/ Central Health Service Officer	Sep 2013 – 15 October 2018
All India Institute of Medical Sciences (AIIMS), Raipur	Pharmacology/Assistant Professor	16 October 2018 – till date

Honors:

- Centum In Physics In Tamilnadu State Board
- Tamilnadu Chief Minister Award during MBBS.
- Cleared and selected in UPSC Combined Medical Services 2012 and posted in Central Health Services under Ministry Of Health and Family Welfare
- Statement of Accomplishment:

- o Antimicrobial Stewardship: Optimization of Antibiotic Practices, Stanford University, December 18, 2013.
- o Genes and the Human Condition (From Behaviour to Biotechnology), University of Maryland, January 20, 2014.

- Got DST SERB young scientist award of international travel grant to attend international conference at Beijing china sep. 18 - 21 2016
- Got Tamilnadu CICS international travel award to attend international conference at Beijing china sep. 18 - 21 2016
- Achievement appreciation in Neyveli Lignite corporation (NLC) in-house journal.

Publications from the Last 3 Years:

[1] Singh, H., S. Ratol, P. Thangaraju, S. Kumar, A. Goel. Pharmacology and Anti-infective Role of Raxibacumab: A Novel Monoclonal Antibody for the Treatment of Anthrax. *West Indian Medical Journal,* DOI is 10.7727/wimj.2015.099.[Pubmed].

[2] Thangaraju, P., T. Selvam, M. K. S. Ali. Metformina, un medicamento antidiabético como agente terapéutico en el tratamiento dele ritema nodoso leproso crónico de moderado a severo Fontilles, *Rev. leprol.,* 479 - 490. [Metformin, an antidiabetic medication as a therapeutic agent in the treatment of moderate to severe chronic leprosy leprosy nodose rhythm Fontilles]

[3] Thangaraju, P., S. Venkatesan, M. K. Showkath Ali. Leprosy case detection campaign (LCDC) for active surveillance *Tropical Doctor,* 0049475517702059.

[4] Michaelsamy, R., P. Thangaraju, V. Gunasekaran, R. Pushpharaj, V. C. Giri, ...Effectiveness of the orientation training for laboratory technicians in leprosy skin smear and nasal smear techniquesin central leprosy teaching and research institute, *India Leprosy Review,* 87 (3), 442 - 447.

[5] Padmalakshmi, P., Y., Shanthi, M., Uma Sekar, Arunagiri, K. Pugazhenthan, T. Phenotypic and Molecular Characterisation of

Carbapenemases in Acinetobacter Species in a Tertiary Care Centre in Tamil Nadu, *India National Journal of Laboratoy Medicine*, 4 (3), 55 - 60.

[6] Thangaraju Pugazhenthan, V. Durai MKSA The role of etanercept in refractory erythema nodosum leprosum. *International Journal of Mycobacteriology.*

[7] Comment on: Blood pressure lowering efficacy of renin inhibitors for primary hypertension, 17, April 2017. *Cochrane Database of Systematic Reviews*. Pugazhenthan Thangaraju.

[8] Thangaraju, P., S. Venkatesan, M. K. Showkath Ali. Screening Needed: Leprosy. *Workplace Health & Safety*, 65 (8), 332 - 332.

[9] Thangaraju, P., S. Venkatesan. Vigilance in Prescribing Nonsteroidal Anti-inflammatory Drugs. *Chinese Medical Journal*, 130 (15), 1889.

[10] Thangaraju, P., S. Venkatesan, A. M. K. Showkath. Leprosy case detection campaign (LCDC) for active surveillance. *Tropical Doctor,* 49475517702059.

[11] Thangaraju, P., S. Venkatesan, A. M. K. Showkath. *Minocycline: A strategy for unresponsive nerve function impairment.* 10.1111/ dth.12535 Dermatologic theraphy.

[12] Pugazhenthan, T., Ravichandran, Aravindan U. et al. (2017). Evaluation of drug use pattern in Central Leprosy Teaching and Research Institute as a Tool to Promote Rational Prescribing. *Indian J. Lepr.,* 89: 99 - 107.

[13] Pugazhenthan, T., Singh, H., Natrajan et al. (2017). Xanthogranulomatous Pyelonephritis Complicated by Emphysematous Pyelonephritis in Lepra Reaction Patient – a Very Rare Occurrence. *Indian J. Lepr.*, 89: 109 - 113.

[14] Goyal, A., H. Singh, V. K. Sehgal, C. R. Jayanthi, R. Munshi, K. L. Bairy, R. Kumar et al. Impact of regulatory spin of pioglitazone on prescription of antidiabetic drugs among physicians in India: A multicentre questionnaire-based observational study. *Indian Journal of Medical Research,* 146 (4), 468.

[15] Pugazhenthan Thangaraju, Sajitha Venkatesan, M. K. Showkath Ali. Final leprosy push: Out of society. *Indian J. Community Med.,* 2018; 43:58 - 9.

[16] Thangaraju, P., Venkatesan, S., Selvan, T. T., Sivshanmugam, E., Showkath, Ali M. K. The resurgence of leprosy in India: Findings from a survey assessing medical professionals' knowledge and preparedness. *Educ. Health Prof.,* 2018; 1:24 - 7.

[17] Thangaraju, P., Venkatesan, S., Sivashanmugam, E., Showkath, Ali M. K. Target Hansen's disease. *J. Family Med. Prim. Care*, 2018; 7(4):838.

[18] Thangaraju, P., Venkatesan, S. Leprosy in Children: Needs for Active Intervention. *Chin. Med. J.,* 2018; 131:1385.

[19] *Nutritional status and morbidity profile of children with contact to leprosy in the rural community.* Yegnaraman Venkatakrishnan, Pugazhenthan Thangaraju, Sathya Jeganathan, Suresh Kumar Sankaran, Rajkumar Kannan. bioRxiv 452995; doi: https://doi.org/10.1101/452995.

[20] Thangaraju, P., Venkatesan, S. News from regulatory corner: Safety communication and recent drug approvals. *Indian J. Drugs Dermatol.,* 2018; 4:45 - 6.

[21] Pugazhenthan, T., Venkatesan, S., Tamilselvan, T. et al. (2018). Information on Drugs Used in Management of Lepra Reactions in Commonly used Drug Information Sources in India. *Indian J. Lepr.,* 90: 129 - 136.

[22] Thangaraju, P., Venkatesan, S., Tamilselvan, T., Sivashanmugam, E., Showkath, Ali M. K. Evaluation of awareness about pharmacovigilance and adverse drug reaction monitoring among medical professionals attending Central Leprosy Institute. *Mustansiriya Med. J.,* 2018; 17:63 - 8.

[23] Thangaraju, P. First mobile application - Lepra reaction basic management guide - Stress on steroids. *Indian J. Drugs Dermatol.*, 2018; 4:85 - 6.

[24] Thangaraju, P., Venkatesan, S., Chadha, V. K. Needs monitoring with quetiapine. *Chin. Med. J.*, 2018; 00:000–000. doi: 10.1097/CM9.0000000000000025.

In: Leprosy: From Diagnosis to Treatment
Editor: Daniel L. Knuth
ISBN: 978-1-53616-629-3

Chapter 5

Association of Vitamin D and the Vitamin D Receptor (VDR) in Leprosy Disease Progression: Implication of New Strategies for Treatment and Clinical Management

Dibyakanti Mandal**, PhD
Department of Biochemistry, PDM University, Haryana, India

Abstract

Leprosy or Hansen's disease is a re-emerging neglected tropical disease caused by *M. leprae*. Most of the leprosy cases have been reported from Indian subcontinent, several tropical countries in Africa and parts of Latin America. In 2017, nearly 200,000 new cases of leprosy were reported and highest prevalence was from India. Multidrug therapy (MDT), consisting of dapsone, rifampicin and clofazimine, is the current recommended treatment for leprosy. Most of the countries across the globe have eliminated leprosy (prevalence is <1 per 10,000). However, emergence of drug-resistant strains and relapse cases are of concern. Therefore, clinical management of leprosy needs implementation of new

* Corresponding Author's E-mail: dkmandal2000@yahoo.com.

strategies. Leprosy is often termed as the 'disease of poor' as the disease is more prevalent among people living with insufficient food and shelter. Vitamin D is a micronutrient and its inadequate intake is associated with many types of health problems including decreased immunity against bacterial and viral infections. Several studies have indicated that vitamin D deficiency is associated with tuberculosis and HIV, though based on current evidences it is inconclusive to say that vitamin D deficiency is the risk factor for prevalence and severity of these diseases. Lower vitamin D level is thought to be associated with leprosy disease as vitamin D is a modulator of Th1, Th2 and toll-like receptor (TLR) signaling and these are the major immune response pathways against *M. leprae*. Also, the countries where vitamin D deficiency is prevalent, the number of leprosy cases is higher and more new cases are reported as compared to the other countries. Vitamin D acts through its receptor VDR, hence VDR is equally important in vitamin D mediated immunity. Recent reports concluded the linkage between low VDR expressions and risk of severe forms of leprosy disease, suggesting that vitamin D and VDR based therapy may be helpful in clinical management of infected individuals and prevent the emergence of new cases. In this chapter we have highlighted the current evidences about the association of vitamin D and VDR to leprosy disease progression, hinting more systematic studies is warranted to better understand the intrinsic pathways involved. The knowledge will help in developing new strategies for treatment and clinical management of leprosy patients.

Keywords: leprosy, *Mycobacterium leprae*, vitamin D, vitamin D receptor

INTRODUCTION

The history of leprosy is thousands of years old. The disease, mainly caused by *Mycobacterium leprae* [2], is also known as Hansen's disease after the name of Dr. Hansen who characterized the disease in the middle of 19th century [1]. *M. leprae* is a gram-positive bacilli and is morphologically similar to *Mycobacterium tuberculosis* (MTb). Worldwide nearly 200,000 cases of leprosy are reported and majority are from India and Brazil. The disease is characterized by skin lesions, muscle weakness, numbness of hands and feet. Leprosy is treatable by drug therapy, but the major concerns are the emergence of new cases because of drug resistance, failure to therapy and missed detection at an early stage [3]. Laboratory diagnosis of *M. leprae* includes slit-skin smear, PCR detection of *M. leprae* gene(s) and these methods are generally accurate [4-7]. Multiplication of the bacteria is very slow, that makes it difficult to grow in culture or in animal models. Armadillos, which are the natural host of the bacteria other than human, are used as animal model for study of leprosy [8, 9].

Multi-drug therapy (MDT) is currently being used to treat leprosy patients. The MDT composes dapsone, refampicin and clofazimine. In case of rifampicin resistance other drugs such as clarithromycin, minocycline or a quinolone are used as second-line treatment [6, 10, 11]. Leprosy disease is associated with poverty, malnutrition and poor living conditions. Deficiency of micronutrients such as zinc, vitamin A, vitamin C and vitamin D is linked to leprosy [12, 13]. Vitamin D is the most studied molecule because of its potential role in immune-modulation and anti-inflammatory function in many diseases and recent evidences suggest that vitamin D level is also associated with leprosy [14]. In this chapter, we have summarized the current knowledge about the role of vitamin D and its receptor VDR in immune-modulation during leprosy disease. The possibility of vitamin D and VDR based therapies for better clinical management of patients and prevention of leprosy disease are also discussed.

Current Epidemiology of Leprosy

Globally 193,118 cases of leprosy are reported from 158 countries in 2017, which is 0.3 cases per 10,000 people worldwide. A total of 211,009 new cases are registered in the same year. Prevalence of leprosy decreased from 5 million in 1983 to <1 cases per 10,000 in 2011 after global leprosy elimination program was introduced. However, new cases are continuously emerging and the new cases are mainly reported from few countries, assumed to be the hotspots. About 90% new cases are reported from only 14 countries across the world. India alone contributes 60% of new cases, whereas Brazil and Indonesia contributes 13% and 8.5% respectively. Remaining new cases are from DRC, Ethiopia, Madagascar, Myanmar, Nepal, Bangladesh and Philippines [15, 16].

In India the prevalence of leprosy is the highest in the world, which includes most of the new cases. Government of India launched the national leprosy eradication program (NLEP) in 2001 aiming to eliminate the disease from the country [11, 15]. The leprosy prevalence rate has been reduced from 4.2 to 0.66 per 10,000 individuals over the period of 2001 to 2011 and met the WHO goal. However, the main concern is the number of emerging new cases every year, which remained unchanged over the last ten years. For example, in 2007 reported new cases were 137,685 and in 2016 the number is 135,485. The data suggests that the natural reservoir is still active and continuously spreading the disease. The failure to diagnose the disease at a very early stage and poor clinical management may be the cause for this [16].

Brazil has the second highest number of leprosy with a total of 25,218 new cases in 2016. The number of new cases in Brazil decreased significantly from 2010 (total 34,894) to 2016, though some parts of Brazil such as central, north and northeastern parts have higher number of new cases as compared to south and southwestern parts. Overall number of cases decreased from 4.71 in 2000 to 1.56 cases per 10,000 in 2010 [17-19].

Indonesia stands third in global leprosy prevalence with close to 17,000 cases in 2017. Though overall prevalence of leprosy decreased since 2000, but the number of new cases remain unchanged most of which are from Java Island [20-22]. Among the other Asian countries, Bangladesh and Nepal have significantly higher number of leprosy cases with continuous reports of new cases from these countries. In African continent, DR Congo, Ethiopia and Nigeria are countries with high prevalence of leprosy.

Immunity in Leprosy

M. leprae enters the body through respiratory route and then spread to other tissues and organs. The pathogen infects skin and nerve cells where the manifestation of the disease can be observed [23, 24]. It is found in the cells of hair follicles, hair shaft, in epidermal cells and both inside and outside of the keratin layers of leprosy patients. Dendritic cells, some of which are phagocytes are also infected with the bacteria and known to migrate to epidermis. Schwann cells (SCs) are the main targets of *M. leprae* and the infection induces demyelination and severe nerve injury [25, 26]. The bacteria infect SCs through binding of PGL-1 glycoprotein present on the surface of the bacteria and laminin-2 on the SCs. Internalization of the pathogen results in bacterial ligation to and activation of neuregulin receptors ErbB2 and Erk1/2 and action of MAP kinase signaling and proliferation leads to demyelination [24, 27, 28].

Leprosy disease is clinically classified within two poles based on histopathology and immunological criteria and these are: tuberculoid polar leprosy (TT), borderline tuberculoid (BT), midboderline (BB), borderline lepromatus (BL) and lepromatous polar leprosy (LL). Leprosy patients are further divided into two categories for treatment purpose: 1) pucibacillary (PB; in case of TT and BT) and 2) multibacillary (MB; in case of BB, BL and LL). This is based on the number of skin lesions present on the patients. If the number of lesion is below 5 then it belongs to PB category and if the number is more than 5 it belongs to MB category [6, 29-34].

Tuberculoid leprosy is classified as inflammatory infiltrate containing well-formed granulomas with differentiated macrophages, epithelioids and predominance of CD4+ T helper cells at the site of infection and with low bacterial index. The lepromatous leprosy is characterized with a preponderance of CD8+T cells at site and absence of granuloma formation. Lepromatous leprosy is generally associated with high bacterial index (BI) at the site of lesion and flattened epidermis. Lepromatous leprosy is associated with Th2 type of immune response with high titer of *M. leprae* antibody and the decreased levels of cell mediated immunity [35, 36]. Leprosy disease progression is associated with inflammation termed as leprosy reactions that result in high degree of morbidity among leprosy patients. They are classified as type I (reversal reaction; RR) or type II (erythema nodosum leprosum; ENL) reactions. Type I reaction occurs in borderline patients (BT, midborderline and BL) whereas ENL only occurs in BL and LL forms. Type I reaction is characterized by edema and erythema of existing skin lesions, the formation of new skin lesions, neuritis, additional sensory and motor loss, and edema of the hands, feet, and face without any systematic symptoms present. Type I reaction is further characterized by the infiltration of $CD4^+$ T cells, differentiated macrophages and thickened epidermis. In contrast, type II reaction is characterized by the appearance of tender, erythematous, subcutaneous nodules located on apparently normal skin, and is associated with systemic symptoms, such as enlarged lymph nodes, fever and edema. Type II or ENL is further characterized by the presence of high levels of pro-inflammatory cytokines such as TNF-α, IL-6, and IL- 1.

BIOLOGY OF VITAMIN D AND VDR

Immune-Modulatory Role of Vitamin D and Its Interaction with Immune Response Pathways in Mycobacterial Diseases

Vitamin D plays major role in calcium homeostasis and bone mineralization and its deficiency causes rickets among children. In addition to its role in calcium absorption, recent studies have demonstrated that active form of vitamin D (1.25 dihydroxy vitamin D or 1.25D) also has important immune-modulatory functions. 1.25D has shown to have potential antimicrobial activity mediated through both acquired and innate immunity and also controls inflammation during infection. Thus 1,25D has a protective role in controlling intercellular growth of *M. leprae* and leprosy disease progression [43-46]. A brief description of immune-modulatory functions of vitamin D is given below.

1,25D induces production of cathelicidin anti-microbial peptide (CAMP) in infected monocytes [47-49]. Cathelicidin is a bacterial cell wall synthesis inhibitor and disrupts phosphatidyl glycerol monolayer. CAMP has multiple VDRE elements (vitamin D receptor elements) on its gene and expression of CAMP is through TLR2 signaling. LL37, a cathelicidin peptide has direct antimicrobial activity and shown to inhibit mycobacterial growth by inducing autophagy through MAPK signaling

[50]. Neutrophils, B cells, T cells, DC also release CAMP and antimicrobial peptides [51-53]. Neutrophils express another class of peptides with antimicrobial activity called defensin (DEFB4), which is also stimulated by 1,25D through VDR activation [54]. Other antimicrobial peptides released from neutrophils are neutrophil peptide 1-3 (HNP1-3) neutrophil gelatinase associated lipocalin (NGAL) [55-57]. Role of 1,25D in expressions of these peptides is yet to be studied.

1,25D regulates the production of Th1 and Th2 cytokines and 1L-17, by which it influences adaptive immunity and inflammation [58-60]. Interestingly, specific T-cell cytokines are able to influence the TLR induced vitamin-D-dependent anti-microbial pathway in human monocytes. The Th1 cytokine IFN-γ enhances the TLR2/1 induction of CYP27B1, cathelicidin and DFEB4. Recent studies have shown a down regulatory effect of 1,25D in activity of cytokine like TNF-α expression in inflammatory disease [61]. The down regulatory effect of 1,25D is not unique to TNF-α expression and was found to decrease the synthesis of IL-2 in activated lymphocytes and also inhibited expression of 1L-1, IL-6 and IL-12 in cultured monocytes and macrophages [62-64]. The ability to suppress *Mycobacterium tuberculosis* (MTb) growth in monocytes has also been linked to the production of bactericidal superoxide anions and to the generation of phagocyte derived reactive oxygen synthesis (NO) [65].

Evidences suggest that 1,25D has anti-inflammatory activity and prevent immunity driven tissue injury in diseases. Anti-inflammatory action of vitamin D include inhibition of IFN-γ, TNF and IL2p40 expressed within the infected PBMCs. 1,25D also inhibits secretion of pro-inflammatory cytokines IL-6, IL-1RA from white blood cells. Supplementation of vitamin D shows increased lymphocyte to monocyte ratio, a marker for healing lesions, also reduction of ESR (erythrocyte sedimentation rate) and CRP (C-reactive protein). These observations suggest that sufficient 1,25D levels help in controlling inflammation at early stages of infections and during disease progression [66-68].

Biosynthesis and Functions of Vitamin D and VDR

The endocrine system of vitamin D is central to the control of bone and calcium homeostasis. D2 and D3 are the two major types of vitamin D. Vitamin D2 is synthesized in plants and fungi, whereas vitamin D3 or calcitriol is produced in relatively large amounts in humans and in majority of vertebrate animals. The active metabolite of vitamin D, 1,25D is involved in calcium and phosphate metabolism and also promotes insulin secretion, innate immunity, and cellular differentiation.

In the presence of UV radiation vitamin D3 is photosynthesized in the skin from 7-dehydrocholesterol and the process involves two steps. First, 7-dehydrocholesterol is photolyzed by ultraviolet light to produce pre-vitamin D3. Second, pre-vitamin D3 spontaneously isomerizes to vitamin D3 (cholecalciferol). Following biosynthesis, inactive vitamin D3 is transported to the proximal tubule of kidney, where it is hydrolyzed to active form 1,25D or calcitriol [69].

The active vitamin D metabolite 1,25D mediates its biological effects by binding to the vitamin D receptor (VDR). The binding of 1,25D to the VDR allows the VDR to act as a transcription factor that modulates the gene expression of transport proteins (such as TRPV6 and calbindin) involved in calcium absorption. Vitamin D deficiency can result in lower bone mineral density and an increased risk of reduced bone density (osteoporosis) or bone fracture. Vitamin D deficiency is a global problem and is associated with poor health and diseases. Limited exposure to sunlight and low intake of vitamin D containing food are among the factors contributing vitamin D deficiency. Generally serum vitamin D level less than 20 ng/ml (<20ng/ml) is termed deficient condition and that between 20ng/ml and 30ng/ml is termed insufficiency. Genetic defects, altered metabolism and external factors also contribute to deficiency. Increased body mass index (BMI), decreased absorption of vitamin D in intestine, increased 1α-hydroxylation of 25(OH)D or increased catabolism of 25(OH)D and 1,25D may lead to deficiency [70, 71]. Deficiency may be caused due to infection or diseases also. Studies have shown that HIV infection causes vitamin D deficiency by altering the levels of cytochrome enzymes that metabolize 1,25D. Certain antiretroviral drugs also induce catabolism of 1,25D and lower the serum levels of active vitamin D [72-76].

Vitamin D Receptor Structure and Properties

Human *VDR* gene is approximately 100 kb long and the pre-mRNA has 14 exons that are distributed through the 5′UTR, coding region and the 3′UTR [77-79]. Multiple promoters within the 5′UTR control the transcription of VDR. Distal and proximal promoters generate multiple VDR transcript variant [77]. Alternative splicing of *VDR* gene also results in VDR transcript variant. The transcript VDR1 lacks an alternate exon in the 5′UTR compared to VDR2, whereas both the variants make the same protein. VDR protein has a nuclear localization motifs and a DNA binding domain with two zinc finger motifs at the N-terminus. Ligand binding domain is present in the C-terminus [80].

The biological action of 1,25D is performed by binding to the receptors VDR and Retinoid X receptor-a (RXR-a) in the nucleus of various cells of the body. VDR is one of the DNA-binding transcription factors but has an important additional property, which it shares only with some other members of nuclear receptor superfamily. Like other members of the human nuclear receptor superfamily, VDR is characterized by a highly conserved DNA binding domain (DBD) and a structurally conserved ligand-binding domain (LBD). This receptor is present in many cells of the immune system including monocytes as well as stimulated macrophages, DCs, natural killer cells and activated B and T cells and it is involved in many processes such as proliferation and differentiation. VDR is activated by macromolecular concentrations of lipophilic molecule, the property that is shared with nuclear receptor for steroid hormones [81]. The ligand-bound VDR activates transcription by hetero-dimerization with RXRs, which is essential for high-affinity DNA binding to cognate vitamin D response elements (VDREs) located in the regulatory regions of 1,25D target genes [82, 83]. Some transcription factors, called ''pioneer factors'' bind regulatory genomic regions at first and start the opening of these loci via the interaction with chromatin modifying enzymes. Ubiquitously expressed transcription factors, such as FOXA1, AP1, SPI1 or SP1, may act as pioneer factors for the VDR [84]. As observed with other transcription factors, the DBD and of VDR cannot contact more than six nucleotides within the major groove of the target DNA and the conserved sequence for VDR binding is RGKTSA (R= A or G, K= G or T and S= C or G), which is also referred to as VDRE or vitamin D response element [85]. Several recent studies using chromatin immune-precipitation assay or ChIP technique have shown there are number of genes that are regulated by VDR. Vitamin D3 stimulation of lymphoblastoma or human monocyte has shown to trigger VDR binding to more than 1500 sites within the genome. The VDR binding site of this gene is located within the intron some 110 kb downstream of transcription start site (TSS) [86].

Numbers of recent studies suggest that VDR maturation is associated with a number of diseases mainly due to defects in immunomodulation. VDR also regulates miRNA (Micro RNA) expression and thus might indirectly involved in key regulation of other genes. VDR regulates expressions of MIR181a MIR-22 and MCM7 gene that encodes MIR106b [87-89]. MicroRNA regulation is linked to several diseases and their presence is sometimes used as marker [90-92].

Association of Vitamin D and VDR with Different Diseases

Vitamin D Deficiency and Diseases

Vitamin D deficiency is a worldwide problem and known to be a risk factor for numerous diseases. The unavailability of standardized methods to assess the vitamin D deficiency makes it difficult to estimate the prevalence of disease correctly. Recent prospective and retrospective studies have shown that individuals with less than 20 ng/ml serum vitamin D levels are at higher risk for colon, prostate and breast cancer [93-97].

VDBP or vitamin D binding protein binds to vitamin D and helps in entry to the cells where it activates gene expression through VDR. Abnormality in VDBP levels in cells is associated to malignancy risk [98].

Diabetes is a worldwide problem and a low vitamin D level is associated with risk of type-2 diabetes among the adults. Based on the available data several hypotheses have been proposed to explain the correlation of vitamin D deficiency and diabetes. Vitamin D is linked to the insulin sensitivity and is associated with insulin resistance of the cell leading to type-2 diabetes. Vitamin D binds the carrier on the surface of islets of beta cells and following entry to the cells it activates many genes through VDR activity. Other studies suggest that in vitamin D deficiency immune and cell signaling pathways are altered which may cause type-2 diabetes [99-101].

High cholesterol levels, smoking, obesity and high blood pressure are the major causes of cardiovascular diseases. Recent studies indicated that vitamin D plays an important role in maintaining normal cardiovascular function. Tissues in cardiovascular system express abundant VDR. Vitamin D suppresses the expression of pro-inflammatory cytokines and also controls oxidative stress through production of NO, thus protect from cardiovascular diseases [102, 103]. Vitamin D is also important in preventing liver diseases. It protects individuals from liver cirrhosis, liver cancer through activation of immune system [104-106].

Young people with HIV/AIDS are at risk for numerous comorbidities typically seen in elderly population, including weakness, metabolic disorder, diabetes, cardiovascular disease and cognitive impairment. Many of these symptoms are associated with vitamin D deficiency. Several recent studies have shown that low vitamin D levels are associated with HIV disease progression and HIV related complications, therefore, understanding the role of vitamin D in preventing HIV associated morbidity and mortality is of particular interest [107-110]. It is known that HIV infection causes vitamin D deficiency by inducing expression of *CYP24B1*.

Antiviral activity of vitamin D is not clearly known and experiments showed replication of R5 and X4 virus in cell type specific manner after vitamin D treatment. Conflicting results showed that vitamin D may be beneficial for the virus replication. HIV and other viruses take different strategies to evade T cell response. Viruses restrict T cell activation by telerogenic status or by T cell exhaustion by T cell overstimulation [80]. Vitamin D treatment can be considered as an immune-modulatory adjuvant in HIV infection. Vitamin D acts as T cell polarization promoting Treg cells that inhibits T effector cells, mainly Th1 [80, 111]. Another concern about using vitamin D as immunosuppressant against HIV infection comes from the expected promotion of T cell exhaustion and viral persistence induced by vitamin D derived cytokine pattern. The molecules in innate immune response pathways such as APOBEC, IFITM family of proteins, defensin molecules restrict HIV-1 replication and the mechanism of inhibition is well studied [112, 113]. It is known that vitamin D stimulates the expression of defensin molecules during MTb infection but there is no such study in HIV infection.

Individuals infected with HIV very often get opportunistic infections by Cryptococcus, Hepatitis B virus (HBV), Hepatitis C virus (HCV) and bacterial diseases other than MTb. Recent literatures have shown that low vitamin D level may be associated to HBV and HCV related health problems and lower vitamin D levels in HIV infection may favor opportunistic infections [114, 115].

VDR and Diseases

The existence of several RFLPs in the *VDR* gene has been described using different restriction enzymes such as Tru9I, TaqI, BsmI, EcoRV and ApaI. Point mutations within the *VDR* gene are the basis of these RFLPs. These mutations lead to transcript and VDR protein variants. Different transcript variants result in altered mRNA stability and splicing pattern which cause different sizes of VDR proteins, altered localization and stability. All these RFLPs are located between the 8 and 9 exons and lay in an area with unknown function. A different case of RFLP is the so-called FokI which results from a T to C change in the exon 2. The change is inside a start codon (ATG), so when the C variant is present, an alternative start site is used leading to a protein with different size. Detailed study was not done to determine the effects of this mutation. The 3′UTR of the *VDR* gene is also a source of several different polymorphisms [116-119].

VDR polymorphisms were shown to be associated with several diseases including cancer and diabetes. Renal failure was found to be linked with certain VDR variants. The complex calcitriol-VDR regulates parathyroid cell proliferation and parathyroid hormone (PTH) synthesis. Thus, the interaction of calcitriol with its receptor inhibits PTH synthesis as well as parathyroid gland cell proliferation. There are reports suggesting that BsmI polymorphism is linked to primary hyperparathyroidism (HPT). There is also report linking the FF genotype of FokI polymorphism with higher PTH levels in pre-dialysis patients [120].

Apart from the effects on bone formation and mineralization, altered calcium handling in the body could lead to different complications, like an increase in absorption and excretion of calcium. BsmI polymorphism with a higher urinary calcium excretion and increased risk of stone formation was reported. Study has shown a decrease in citrate urinary excretion among the individuals with the bb phenotype, confirming the theory of a higher risk of kidney stones in the population presenting the VDR allele [121].

An association has been described between 1,25D and susceptibility to and outcome of some cancers, like breast, prostate and colon cancers. Studies suggest the relationship between the polyA polymorphism of the *VDR* gene (one of the UTR polymorphisms) and prostate cancer in the US population. VDR TaqI polymorphism and an increased risk of prostate cancer were observed [97, 122-128].

The involvement of VDR has been suggested in the etiology of both independent and dependent Diabetes Mellitus (DM). *VDR* gene polymorphisms are likely to be related to T-cell mediated autoimmune disease thus affects clinical outcome of DM. In type 1 DM, BsmI polymorphism has been linked to susceptibility to present the disease among people from different regions. Following the same pattern ApaI,

TaqI and FokI were found associated to type 2 DM in some reports [129-131].

ASSOCIATION OF VITAMIN D AND VDR WITH LEPROSY AND *MYCOBACTERIAL* INFECTIONS

According to recent WHO report more than 95% leprosy cases are from 14 countries. Geographically these are tropical countries and a higher prevalence of vitamin D deficiency among general population was reported from these places. Table 1 shows the data from five countries with higher number of leprosy cases and percentage of vitamin D insufficiency or deficiency among the general population. The data suggests a correlation between vitamin D status and leprosy disease prevalence.

Table 1. Prevalence of vitamin D insufficiency in five countries with highest rate of leprosy prevalence and highest number of new cases

Country Name	Leprosy prevalence IN 2017	New cases in 2018	Vitamin insufficiency
India	88166	134184	>90%
Brazil	22710	38914	77%
Indonesia	18248	17441	>50%
Bangladesh	3132	5249	36%
Nepal	2559	4708	73%

Both *M. leprae* and *M. tuberculosis* are gram-positive bacilli and have similarities in terms of pathogenesis and immune response pathways, so pattern of immune-modulatory and antimicrobial effects exerted by vitamin D are expected to be similar for both the pathogens. Very limited data is available about the vitamin D levels among the leprosy patients to demonstrate the correlation between vitamin D deficiency and leprosy. One study from Kolkata, India has shown low vitamin D levels among the leprosy patients. Another study from North India also showed low vitamin D among leprosy patients [132, 133]. A recent study from Indonesia have shown association of multibacillary leprosy (more complex form of the disease), with vitamin D deficiency [134]. More systematic studies are to be conducted to generate adequate data for establishing the role of vitamin D in leprosy.

Antimicrobial activities of vitamin D against mycobacteria were studied in detail in MTb infections. Recent studies have shown that vitamin D levels are low among tuberculosis patients compared to healthy individuals [73, 135, 136]. Higher prevalence of low serum 1,25D levels among TB patients were found in Asian and African countries [137, 138]. Two possible conclusions can be drawn from this data: first, individuals with vitamin D deficiency are more susceptible to MTb infection. Second, *M. tuberculosis* infection causes vitamin D deficiency in patients.. Evidences suggest that abundant vitamin D helps in preventing spread of MTb and also plays important role in clearing of the pathogen by modulating the immune response pathways and through direct antimicrobial activities.

Exact mechanism how 1,25D mediates immune activation to fight MTb infection is not clear yet. However, studies have indicated that the immune response can be triggered even with insufficient levels of 1,25D but immune response gets activated only at adequate levels of 1,25D. IFN-γ, which plays central role in providing immune response against the TB bacteria, also requires sufficient levels of 1,25D to be effective. Also, 1,25D modulates monocytes and macrophage activity in the body and plays a role in human innate immunity to certain infectious agents like MTb [50, 136, 139, 140]. A possible mechanism for this is enhanced fusion of phagosome and lysosome in infected macrophages as evidenced by the capacity of MTb to prevent macrophage maturation and phagolysosome formation, which is reversed in the presence of 1,25D. 1,25D induces production of LL-37, an antimicrobial peptide of cathelicidin family that inhibits infectious microbes including MTb [135-137, 139, 141]. A recent study reported that vitamin D has a metabolic role in MTb growth, showing that vitamin D treatment of MTb infected macrophages abrogated infection-induced accumulation of lipid droplets, which are absolutely necessary for *M. tuberculosis* growth. Further investigation revealed that 1,25D down-regulates the pro-adipogenic peroxisome activated receptor gamma in infected macrophages [142].

Role of vitamin D receptor (VDR) in leprosy disease was not assessed until recently. In a small study among the leprosy patients from Kolkata, India it was shown that leprosy patients with type-I or type-II reaction have low levels of vitamin D in serum. Interestingly, individuals with type II reaction associated with neuritis/ENL have very low VDR mRNA expression levels ranging from 5% to 10% only to that of the healthy control samples. This is the first report implicating that VDR expression levels may determine the complexity and severity of leprosy disease progression [133]. Low VDR expression may be due to multiple mutations in coding or non-coding regions of VDR. Another study from north India also reported low VDR expression among leprosy patients [132]. One recent study from Indonesia suggested that significantly low serum VDR is associated with leprosy disease [143].

Certain VDR genotypes were found to be associated with leprosy. In tuberculoid leprosy, the tt genotype was found at significantly higher frequency than in the controls. In contrast, the TT genotype was found at increased frequency in the lepromatous leprosy group compared with the controls. Heterozygotes of genotype Tt were found less frequently in both leprosy types than in controls [144]. The association between VDR genotype and lepromatous leprosy provides further evidence supporting the role of vitamin D receptor as an immune response gene regulator causing susceptibility to infection. The mechanism remains unclear but may relate to the increased differentiation and cytotoxicity observed in macrophages treated with 1,25D3. Type 2 leprosy reaction, which is associated with low VDR, may have altered TNF-α mediated immune response. Such in vitro studies are not possible *In-vitro* studies for *M. leprae* are not possible, but early studies of the treatment of leprosy with medications containing vitamin D are consistent with a possible immune-modulatory effect on this bacterium.

ROLE OF BRONCHOALVEOLAR LAVAGE FLUID (BALF) VITAMIN D IN LEPROSY

M. leprae enters body through respiratory route and BAL macrophages are the first immune cells that the pathogen encounters. Alveolar macrophages have defensive role with phagocytic and antigen processing functions. Thus level of immune protection provided by BAL macrophages determine the extent of spread of *M. leprae* to other tissues and organs. Vitamin D in BALF mediates activation of immune response exerted by macrophages and provide protection against invading pathogens including *M. leprae*.

Alveolar macrophages (AMs) are primary effector cells in the host response to a pathogen. MTb infection in mouse model showed that airway macrophages are involved in spread of the bacteria in other tissues through fusion of phagosome and lysosome. Recent studies conducted among HIV-1 infected individuals showed that BAL macrophages in infected individuals have low phagocytic activity, impaired TNF-α release and the exogenous vitamin D can partially rescue TNF-α release [140]. A separate study reported that BAL vitamin D levels in HIV-1 infected individuals are lower compared to uninfected subjects, which is in agreement with the earlier reports showing that HIV infection decreases vitamin D levels [138]. As both MTb and *M. leprae* have similar mode of pathogenesis, it is assumed that vitamin D in BALF also plays important role in preventing *M. leprae* multiplication and leprosy disease progression.

In addition to the BALF vitamin D levels, it is presumed that altered VDR expressions will also have the similar effects on immune response against pathogens. It is important to look for VDR expression levels in BAL macrophages along with the estimation of vitamin D levels among the individuals at risk of leprosy and mycobacterial diseases. So far no animal study or ex vivo study has been conducted to determine role of BAL macrophages in *M. leprae* infection under the conditions of vitamin D deficiency or with defect in VDR expression. Also, no information is available regarding the status of BAL vitamin D levels among leprosy patients.

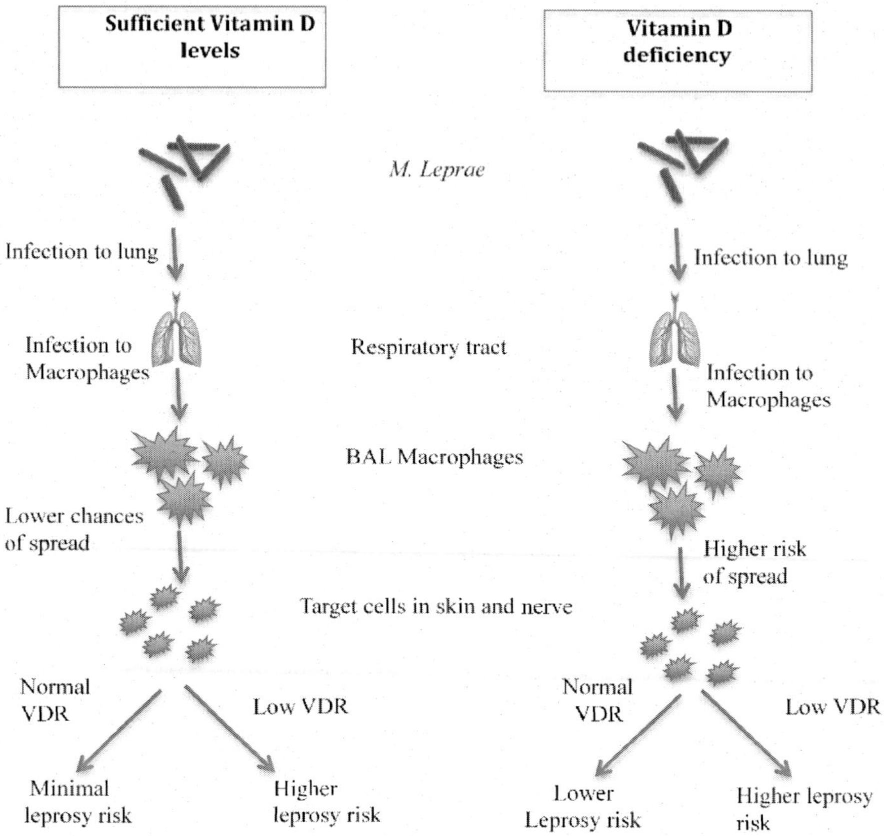

Figure 1. The figure illustrates the role of vitamin D and VDR in leprosy. *M. leprae* invades human via respiratory route. The bacteria infect alveolar macrophages and then spread to other tissues like skin and nerve by unknown mechanism. In presence of abundant vitamin D and VDR, macrophages and other immune cells in lung are able to restrict spread of *M. leprae* and there is a lower chance of leprosy. In case of normal vitamin D levels but decreased VDR level the risk of leprosy is higher. In case of vitamin D deficiency and low VDR there is always higher risk of leprosy and there is chance of more severe and complex disease progression.

In Figure 1, we have summarized the predicted role of vitamin D and VDR in both BALF and serum in controlling *M. leprae* infection and lowering risk of leprosy. Among individuals with normal vitamin D and VDR levels, *M. leprae* entry from respiratory tract to other tissue is restricted. Abundant vitamin D and VDR also prevents intracellular bacterium growth and provide immune protection and there is minimum risk of leprosy. In individuals with vitamin D deficiency or due to low VDR levels susceptibility to *M. laprae* infection is more and there is a higher risk of severe forms of leprosy disease.

VITAMIN D AND VDR BASED THERAPIES FOR CLINICAL MANAGEMENT OF LEPROSY

Vitamin D deficiency is very common worldwide with some geographical variations. Vitamin D deficiency makes an individual susceptible to diseases and infection, disease complexity and severity. Therefore vitamin D supplementation may be an effective way to prevent diseases and quick recovery from sickness. In recent past several clinical trials have been conducted to measure the effects of vitamin D supplementation among the TB and HIV/TB infected individuals undergoing treatment for TB and HIV. Significant benefits however were not observed from these trials and several explanations were given, these include supplementation of vitamin D along with MDT, doses of vitamin D and duration of supplementation. More studies are required to gather sufficient evidence to conclude about the true benefits.

Poverty, malnutrition, poor intake of vitamin D are the risk factors of leprosy and limited studies have shown that there is a prevalence of lower vitamin D levels among leprosy patients [132, 133]. Therefore vitamin D supplementation could be an effective measure for better clinical management of the disease and in controlling the spread of the *M. leprae*.. Effective strategies are to be designed for a successful supplementation program.

In addition to vitamin D, VDR is also important in regulating the expressions of genes of immune system. So, optimum level of VDR expression is required for its function. .Three recent studies mentioned that leprosy disease severity and complexity is closely associated with cellular VDR levels. Low VDR expression levels in cells may be due to genetic defects caused by mutations that lead to truncated proteins, unstable mRNA and their incorrect localization [132, 133]. Individuals with normal

Vitamin D levels in body but have a defective *VDR gene* are thus susceptible to diseases. This implicates that the level of vitamin D, expression of its receptor (VDR) are to be monitored. In case of defects in VDR, gene therapy is an option. Transgene expression or correction of mutated genes through gene targeting could be effective ways to restore the VDR function. Sometimes altered VDR structure may prevent efficient vitamin D binding to VDR and vitamin D mediated immune response is inhibited due to weak vitamin D-VDR interaction. Designing and use of vitamin D analogues in such cases may help in activating immune system in diseases including leprosy. These analogues have been recently tested for their function as immune modulator alternative to vitamin D [145-148].

Conclusion

Vitamin D sufficiency contributes to better health and immunity to different diseases including cancer, diabetes and infection. Line of evidences suggests that vitamin D deficiency is linked to mycobacterial diseases including leprosy. Vitamin D is associated with leprosy disease progression, reaction complexity and activation of immune response. BAL vitamin D helps in preventing spread of *M. leprae* to other tissues by stimulating antimicrobial activities of alveolar macrophages, whereas serum vitamin D mediates the clearance of the bacteria from circulating blood cells and infected tissues by increasing phagocytic activity of macrophages and boosting the innate immunity. Vitamin D acts through its receptor VDR that upon binding to vitamin D induces expression of number of genes of immune system, thus VDR plays equally important role in controlling the infection.

Current leprosy elimination program is focusing on early diagnosis of leprosy to prevent new cases and also looking to reduce the number of relapse and drug resistant cases. Looking at the benefits of vitamin D in multiple steps during *M. leprae* replication, it is strongly suggested to incorporate vitamin D based therapy along with antimicrobial drug regimen. At first, the program should include regular monitoring of vitamin D status of individuals from each household in the pandemic region particularly people living with the leprosy patients. If deficiency is found they should be advised for vitamin D supplementation. Large scale studies should be conducted in these affected areas and the objectives will be to determine 1) the proportion of individuals with vitamin D deficiency; 2) the benefits of vitamin D supplementation; 3) to determine the vitamin D binding protein (VDBP) and VDR levels and 4) to determine VDR genotype.

Vitamin D supplementation is a cheap and effective way. India has more than 60% of global leprosy cases and there are 50-90% people living with vitamin D deficiency. The prevalence is high among the elderly people, pregnant and menopausal women At present India does not have such policy, but Govt. of India is making rapid headways towards the introduction of vitamin D supplementation through food fortification. Food fortification in USA and Canada resulted in improved vitamin status among the general population but long term benefit from this is yet to be determined before India adopts the food fortification policy. Furthermore, vitamin D deficiency is individual specific and food fortification program to be implemented should be within the threshold limit and may be done according to the country's food and drug administration guidelines.

In future, effort in determining the importance of VDR expression levels and VDR polymorphisms with different types of leprosy is warranted. VDR based gene therapy will be a novel approach in order to reduce the burden of leprosy and other diseases. Designing of vitamin D analogues and using them as substitutes in vitamin D deficiency may be an effective approach to combat leprosy. Vitamin D based therapy in combination with MDT is predicted to be a successful way to reduce the burden of leprosy.

REFERENCES

[1] Suzuki K, Akama T, Kawashima A, Yoshihara A, Yotsu RR, Ishii N: Current status of leprosy: epidemiology, basic science and

clinical perspectives. *The Journal of dermatology* 2012, 39(2):121-129.

[2] *Leprosy fact sheet* (revised in February 2010). Releve epidemiologique hebdomadaire 2009, 85(6):46-48.

[3] Matsuoka M: [Review of sentinel surveillance for drug resistance in leprosy conducted by WHO Global Leprosy Programme]. Nihon Hansenbyo Gakkai zasshi = *Japanese journal of leprosy: official organ of the Japanese Leprosy Association* 2011, 80(1):71-77.

[4] Bhushan P, Sardana K, Koranne RV, Choudhary M, Manjul P: Diagnosing multibacillary leprosy: a comparative evaluation of diagnostic accuracy of slit-skin smear, bacterial index of granuloma and WHO operational classification. *Indian journal of dermatology, venereology and leprology* 2008, 74(4):322-326.

[5] Alemu Belachew W, Naafs B: Position statement: LEPROSY: Diagnosis, treatment and follow-up. *Journal of the European Academy of Dermatology and Venereology: JEADV* 2019, 33 (7):1205-1213.

[6] Aamir M, Sadaf A, Khan S, Perveen S, Khan A: Recent Advancement in the Diagnosis and Treatment of Leprosy. *Current topics in medicinal chemistry* 2018, 18(18):1550-1558.

[7] 7.Pathak VK, Singh I, Turankar RP, Lavania M, Ahuja M, Singh V, Sengupta U: Utility of multiplex PCR for early diagnosis and household contact surveillance for leprosy. *Diagnostic microbiology and infectious disease* 2019.

[8] Job CK: Nine-banded armadillo (*Dasypus novemcinctus*) as an animal model for leprosy. *Indian journal of leprosy* 1991, 63(3-4):356-361.

[9] Storrs EE, Binford CH, Migaki G: Animal model of human disease: lepromatous leprosy. *The American journal of pathology* 1978, 92(3):813-816.

[10] [New WHO recommendations for the treatment of leprosy]. *Acta leprologica* 1997, 10(4):189.

[11] Kumar A, Girdhar A, Chakma JK, Girdhar BK: WHO multidrug therapy for leprosy: epidemiology of default in treatment in Agra

district, Uttar Pradesh, India. *BioMed research international* 2015, 2015:705804.

[12] Rao KN, Saha K, Chakrabarty AK: Undernutrition and lepromatous leprosy. III. Micronutrients and their transport proteins. *Human nutrition Clinical nutrition* 1987, 41(2):127-134.

[13] Passos Vazquez CM, Mendes Netto RS, Ferreira Barbosa KB, Rodrigues de Moura T, de Almeida RP, Duthie MS, Ribeiro de Jesus A: Micronutrients influencing the immune response in leprosy. *Nutricion hospitalaria* 2014, 29(1):26-36.

[14] Lu'o'ng K, Nguyen LT: Role of the vitamin D in leprosy. *The American journal of the medical sciences* 2012, 343(6):471-482.

[15] Rao PS: Current epidemiology of leprosy in India. *Leprosy review* 2006, 77(4):292-294.

[16] Arif T, Amin SS, Adil M, Dorjay K, Raj D: Leprosy in the post-elimination era: a clinico-epidemiological study from a northern Indian tertiary care hospital. *Acta dermatovenerologica Alpina, Pannonica, et Adriatica* 2019, 28(1):7-10.

[17] Cunha C, Pedrosa VL, Dias LC, Braga A, Chrusciak-Talhari A, Santos M, Penna GO, Talhari S, Talhari C: A historical overview of leprosy epidemiology and control activities in Amazonas, Brazil. *Revista da Sociedade Brasileira de Medicina Tropical* 2015, 48 Suppl 1:55-62.

[18] Rosa PS, D'Espindula HRS, Melo ACL, Fontes ANB, Finardi AJ, Belone AFF, Sartori BGC, Pires CAA, Soares CT, Marques FB et al: Emergence and transmission of drug/multidrug-resistant *Mycobacterium leprae* in a former leprosy colony in the Brazilian Amazon. *Clinical infectious diseases: an official publication of the Infectious Diseases Society of America* 2019.

[19] Brito AL, Monteiro LD, Ramos Junior AN, Heukelbach J, Alencar CH: Temporal trends of leprosy in a Brazilian state capital in Northeast Brazil: epidemiology and analysis by joinpoints, 2001 to 2012. *Revista brasileira de epidemiologia = Brazilian journal of epidemiology* 2016, 19(1):194-204.

[20] Bakker MI, Hatta M, Kwenang A, Klatser PR, Oskam L: Epidemiology of leprosy on five isolated islands in the Flores Sea, Indonesia. *Tropical medicine & international health: TM & IH* 2002, 7(9):780-787.

[21] Progress in leprosy control: Indonesia, 1991-2008. *Releve epidemiologique hebdomadaire* 2010, 85(26):249-262.

[22] Tosepu R, Gunawan J, Effendy DS, Fadmi FR: Stigma and increase of leprosy cases in South East Sulawesi Province, Indonesia. *African health sciences* 2018, 18(1):29-31.

[23] Davey TF: New dimensions in our understanding of the transmission of leprosy and their impact on priorities in leprosy control. *Leprosy in India* 1980, 52(1):104-113.

[24] Bhat RM, Prakash C: Leprosy: an overview of pathophysiology. *Interdisciplinary perspectives on infectious diseases* 2012, 2012: 181089.

[25] Mukherjee R, Antia NH: Intracellular multiplication of leprosy-derived mycobacteria in Schwann cells of dorsal root ganglion cultures. *Journal of clinical microbiology* 1985, 21(5):808-814.

[26] Spierings E, De Boer T, Zulianello L, Ottenhoff TH: The role of Schwann cells, T cells and *Mycobacterium leprae* in the immunopathogenesis of nerve damage in leprosy. *Leprosy review* 2000, 71 Suppl:S121-129.

[27] Andrade PR, Jardim MR, da Silva AC, Manhaes PS, Antunes SL, Vital R, Prata RB, Petito RB, Pinheiro RO, Sarno EN: Inflammatory Cytokines Are Involved in Focal Demyelination in Leprosy Neuritis. *Journal of neuropathology and experimental neurology* 2016, 75(3):272-283.

[28] Tapinos N, Ohnishi M, Rambukkana A: ErbB2 receptor tyrosine kinase signaling mediates early demyelination induced by leprosy bacilli. *Nature medicine* 2006, 12(8):961-966.

[29] Murthy PK: Clinical manifestations, diagnosis and classification of leprosy. *Journal of the Indian Medical Association* 2004, 102 (12):678-679.

[30] Bhatia AS, Katoch K, Narayanan RB, Ramu G, Mukherjee A, Lavania RK: Clinical and histopathological correlation in the classification of leprosy. *International journal of leprosy and other mycobacterial diseases: official organ of the International Leprosy Association* 1993, 61(3):433-438.

[31] Saigawa K: [Leprosy control by WHO. 4. Classification of the disease]. *Repura Leprosy* 1973, 42(2):176-177.

[32] Eichelmann K, Gonzalez Gonzalez SE, Salas-Alanis JC, Ocampo-Candiani J: Leprosy. An update: definition, pathogenesis, classification, diagnosis, and treatment. *Actas dermo-sifiliograficas* 2013, 104(7):554-563.

[33] Sehgal VN, Jain MK, Srivastava G: Evolution of the classification of leprosy. *International journal of dermatology* 1989, 28(3):161-167.

[34] Parkash O: Classification of leprosy into multibacillary and paucibacillary groups: an analysis. *FEMS immunology and medical microbiology* 2009, 55(1):1-5.

[35] Walker SL, Lockwood DN: The clinical and immunological features of leprosy. *British medical bulletin* 2006, 77-78:103-121.

[36] Walker SL, Lockwood DN: Leprosy. *Clinics in dermatology* 2007, 25(2):165-172.

[37] Walker SL, Lockwood DN: Leprosy type 1 (reversal) reactions and their management. *Leprosy review* 2008, 79(4):372-386.

[38] Modlin RL: Th1-Th2 paradigm: insights from leprosy. *The Journal of investigative dermatology* 1994, 102(6):828-832.

[39] Modlin RL: The innate immune response in leprosy. *Current opinion in immunology* 2010, 22(1):48-54.

[40] Andrade PR, Pinheiro RO, Sales AM, Illarramendi X, Barbosa MG, Moraes MO, Jardim MR, Nery JA, Sampaio EP, Sarno EN: Type 1 reaction in leprosy: a model for a better understanding of tissue immunity under an immunopathological condition. *Expert review of clinical immunology* 2015, 11(3):391-407.

[41] Lockwood DN, Lucas SB, Desikan KV, Ebenezer G, Suneetha S, Nicholls P: The histological diagnosis of leprosy type 1 reactions: identification of key variables and an analysis of the process of

histological diagnosis. *Journal of clinical pathology* 2008, 61(5):595-600.

[42] Yamamura M: Defining protective responses to pathogens: cytokine profiles in leprosy lesions. *Science* 1992, 255(5040):12.

[43] Gatti D, Idolazzi L, Fassio A: Vitamin D: not just bone, but also immunity. *Minerva medica* 2016, 107(6):452-460.

[44] Bartley J: Vitamin D: emerging roles in infection and immunity. *Expert review of anti-infective therapy* 2010, 8(12):1359-1369.

[45] Park K, Elias PM, Oda Y, Mackenzie D, Mauro T, Holleran WM, Uchida Y: Regulation of cathelicidin antimicrobial peptide expression by an endoplasmic reticulum (ER) stress signaling, vitamin D receptor-independent pathway. *The Journal of biological chemistry* 2011, 286(39):34121-34130.

[46] De Luca P, de Girolamo L, Perucca Orfei C, Vigano M, Cecchinato R, Brayda-Bruno M, Colombini A: Vitamin D's Effect on the Proliferation and Inflammation of Human Intervertebral Disc Cells in Relation to the Functional Vitamin D Receptor Gene FokI Polymorphism. *International journal of molecular sciences* 2018, 19(7).

[47] Gombart AF: The vitamin D-antimicrobial peptide pathway and its role in protection against infection. *Future microbiology* 2009, 4(9):1151-1165.

[48] White JH: Vitamin D as an inducer of cathelicidin antimicrobial peptide expression: past, present and future. *The Journal of steroid biochemistry and molecular biology* 2010, 121(1-2):234-238.

[49] Albenali LH, Danby S, Moustafa M, Brown K, Chittock J, Shackley F, Cork MJ: Vitamin D and antimicrobial peptide levels in patients with atopic dermatitis and atopic dermatitis complicated by eczema herpeticum: A pilot study. *The Journal of allergy and clinical immunology* 2016, 138(6):1715-1719 e1714.

[50] Yamshchikov AV, Kurbatova EV, Kumari M, Blumberg HM, Ziegler TR, Ray SM, Tangpricha V: Vitamin D status and antimicrobial peptide cathelicidin (LL-37) concentrations in patients

with active pulmonary tuberculosis. *The American journal of clinical nutrition* 2010, 92(3):603-611.

[51] Hansdottir S, Monick MM, Hinde SL, Lovan N, Look DC, Hunninghake GW: Respiratory epithelial cells convert inactive vitamin D to its active form: potential effects on host defense. *Journal of immunology* 2008, 181(10):7090-7099.

[52] Di Nardo A, Vitiello A, Gallo RL: Cutting edge: mast cell antimicrobial activity is mediated by expression of cathelicidin antimicrobial peptide. *Journal of immunology* 2003, 170(5):2274-2278.

[53] Agerberth B, Charo J, Werr J, Olsson B, Idali F, Lindbom L, Kiessling R, Jornvall H, Wigzell H, Gudmundsson GH: The human antimicrobial and chemotactic peptides LL-37 and alpha-defensins are expressed by specific lymphocyte and monocyte populations. *Blood* 2000, 96(9):3086-3093.

[54] De Filippis A, Fiorentino M, Guida L, Annunziata M, Nastri L, Rizzo A: Vitamin D reduces the inflammatory response by *Porphyromonas gingivalis* infection by modulating human beta-defensin-3 in human gingival epithelium and periodontal ligament cells. *International immunopharmacology* 2017, 47:106-117.

[55] Bunz H, Weyrich P, Peter A, Baumann D, Tschritter O, Guthoff M, Beck R, Jahn G, Artunc F, Haring HU et al: Urinary Neutrophil Gelatinase-Associated Lipocalin (NGAL) and proteinuria predict severity of acute kidney injury in Puumala virus infection. *BMC infectious diseases* 2015, 15:464.

[56] Tarazi YH, Khalifeh MS, Abu Al-Kebash MM, Gharaibeh MH: Neutrophil gelatinase-associated lipocalin (NGAL) and insulin-like growth factor (IGF)-1 association with a *Mannheimia haemolytica* infection in sheep. *Veterinary immunology and immunopathology* 2014, 161(3-4):151-160.

[57] Oppenheim JJ, Biragyn A, Kwak LW, Yang D: Roles of antimicrobial peptides such as defensins in innate and adaptive immunity. *Annals of the rheumatic diseases* 2003, 62 Suppl 2:ii17-21.

[58] Boonstra A, Barrat FJ, Crain C, Heath VL, Savelkoul HF, O'Garra A: 1alpha,25-Dihydroxyvitamin d3 has a direct effect on naive CD4(+) T cells to enhance the development of Th2 cells. *Journal of immunology* 2001, 167(9):4974-4980.

[59] Tang J, Zhou R, Luger D, Zhu W, Silver PB, Grajewski RS, Su SB, Chan CC, Adorini L, Caspi RR: Calcitriol suppresses antiretinal autoimmunity through inhibitory effects on the Th17 effector response. *Journal of immunology* 2009, 182(8):4624-4632.

[60] Du T, Zhou ZG, You S, Huang G, Lin J, Yang L, Li X, Zhou WD, Chao C: Modulation of monocyte hyperresponsiveness to TLR ligands by 1,25-dihydroxy-vitamin D3 from LADA and T2DM. *Diabetes research and clinical practice* 2009, 83(2):208-214.

[61] Ojaimi S, Skinner NA, Strauss BJ, Sundararajan V, Woolley I, Visvanathan K: Vitamin D deficiency impacts on expression of toll-like receptor-2 and cytokine profile: a pilot study. *Journal of translational medicine* 2013, 11:176.

[62] Calton EK, Keane KN, Newsholme P, Soares MJ: The Impact of Vitamin D Levels on Inflammatory Status: A Systematic Review of Immune Cell Studies. *PloS one* 2015, 10(11):e0141770.

[63] Pojednic RM, Ceglia L, Lichtenstein AH, Dawson-Hughes B, Fielding RA: Vitamin D receptor protein is associated with interleukin-6 in human skeletal muscle. *Endocrine* 2015, 49(2):512-520.

[64] Heine G, Niesner U, Chang HD, Steinmeyer A, Zugel U, Zuberbier T, Radbruch A, Worm M: 1,25-dihydroxyvitamin D(3) promotes IL-10 production in human B cells. *European journal of immunology* 2008, 38(8):2210-2218.

[65] Onwuneme C, Blanco A, O'Neill A, Watson B, Molloy EJ: Vitamin D enhances reactive oxygen intermediates production in phagocytic cells in term and preterm infants. *Pediatric research* 2016, 79(4):654-661.

[66] Richmond BW, Drake WP: Vitamin D, innate immunity, and sarcoidosis granulomatous inflammation: insights from

mycobacterial research. *Current opinion in pulmonary medicine* 2010, 16(5):461-464.

[67] Nguyen VT, Li X, Elli EF, Ayloo SM, Castellanos KJ, Fantuzzi G, Freels S, Braunschweig CL: Vitamin D, inflammation, and relations to insulin resistance in premenopausal women with morbid obesity. *Obesity* 2015, 23(8):1591-1597.

[68] Mangin M, Sinha R, Fincher K: Inflammation and vitamin D: the infection connection. *Inflammation research: official journal of the European Histamine Research Society* [et al.] 2014, 63(10):803-819.

[69] Berdal A: [Vitamin D: biosynthesis, metabolism and mechanism of action at the cellular level]. *Journal de biologie buccale* 1992, 20(2):71-83.

[70] Bikle DD: Vitamin D insufficiency/deficiency in gastrointestinal disorders. *Journal of bone and mineral research: the official journal of the American Society for Bone and Mineral Research* 2007, 22 Suppl 2:V50-54.

[71] Wortsman J, Matsuoka LY, Chen TC, Lu Z, Holick MF: Decreased bioavailability of vitamin D in obesity. *The American journal of clinical nutrition* 2000, 72(3):690-693.

[72] Pinzone MR, Di Rosa M, Celesia BM, Condorelli F, Malaguarnera M, Madeddu G, Martellotta F, Castronuovo D, Gussio M, Coco C et al: LPS and HIV gp120 modulate monocyte/macrophage CYP27B1 and CYP24A1 expression leading to vitamin D consumption and hypovitaminosis D in HIV-infected individuals. *European review for medical and pharmacological sciences* 2013, 17(14):1938-1950.

[73] Liu PT, Stenger S, Li H, Wenzel L, Tan BH, Krutzik SR, Ochoa MT, Schauber J, Wu K, Meinken C et al. Toll-like receptor triggering of a vitamin D-mediated human antimicrobial response. *Science* 2006, 311(5768):1770-1773.

[74] Brodie MJ, Boobis AR, Hillyard CJ, Abeyasekera G, MacIntyre I, Park BK: Effect of isoniazid on vitamin D metabolism and hepatic monooxygenase activity. *Clinical pharmacology and therapeutics* 1981, 30(3):363-367.

[75] Brodie MJ, Boobis AR, Dollery CT, Hillyard CJ, Brown DJ, Macintyre I, Park BK: Rifampicin and vitamin D metabolism in man [proceedings]. *British journal of clinical pharmacology* 1980, 9(3):286P-287P.

[76] Cozzolino M, Vidal M, Arcidiacono MV, Tebas P, Yarasheski KE, Dusso AS: HIV-protease inhibitors impair vitamin D bioactivation to 1,25-dihydroxyvitamin D. *Aids* 2003, 17(4):513-520.

[77] Crofts LA, Hancock MS, Morrison NA, Eisman JA: Multiple promoters direct the tissue-specific expression of novel N-terminal variant human vitamin D receptor gene transcripts. *Proceedings of the National Academy of Sciences of the United States of America* 1998, 95(18):10529-10534.

[78] Baker AR, McDonnell DP, Hughes M, Crisp TM, Mangelsdorf DJ, Haussler MR, Pike JW, Shine J, O'Malley BW: Cloning and expression of full-length cDNA encoding human vitamin D receptor. *Proceedings of the National Academy of Sciences of the United States of America* 1988, 85(10):3294-3298.

[79] Miyamoto K, Kesterson RA, Yamamoto H, Taketani Y, Nishiwaki E, Tatsumi S, Inoue Y, Morita K, Takeda E, Pike JW: Structural organization of the human vitamin D receptor chromosomal gene and its promoter. *Molecular endocrinology* 1997, 11(8):1165-1179.

[80] Caruz JFaA: Vitamin D and HIV infection: Banthem Science Publisher; 2010.

[81] Molnar F, Perakyla M, Carlberg C: Vitamin D receptor agonists specifically modulate the volume of the ligand-binding pocket. *The Journal of biological chemistry* 2006, 281(15):10516-10526.

[82] Mangelsdorf DJ, Thummel C, Beato M, Herrlich P, Schutz G, Umesono K, Blumberg B, Kastner P, Mark M, Chambon P et al: The nuclear receptor superfamily: the second decade. *Cell* 1995, 83(6):835-839.

[83] Nagy L, Schwabe JW: Mechanism of the nuclear receptor molecular switch. *Trends in biochemical sciences* 2004, 29(6):317-324.

[84] Schule R, Umesono K, Mangelsdorf DJ, Bolado J, Pike JW, Evans RM: Jun-Fos and receptors for vitamins A and D recognize a

common response element in the human osteocalcin gene. *Cell* 1990, 61(3):497-504.

[85] Carlberg C, Bendik I, Wyss A, Meier E, Sturzenbecker LJ, Grippo JF, Hunziker W: Two nuclear signalling pathways for vitamin D. *Nature* 1993, 361(6413):657-660.

[86] Pike JW, Meyer MB: The vitamin D receptor: new paradigms for the regulation of gene expression by 1,25-dihydroxyvitamin D(3). *Endocrinology and metabolism clinics of North America* 2010, 39(2):255-269, table of contents.

[87] Duggal J, Harrison JS, Studzinski GP, Wang X: Involvement of microRNA181a in differentiation and cell cycle arrest induced by a plant-derived antioxidant carnosic acid and vitamin D analog doxercalciferol in human leukemia cells. *MicroRNA* 2012, 1(1):26-33.

[88] Alvarez-Diaz S, Valle N, Ferrer-Mayorga G, Lombardia L, Herrera M, Dominguez O, Segura MF, Bonilla F, Hernando E, Munoz A: MicroRNA-22 is induced by vitamin D and contributes to its antiproliferative, antimigratory and gene regulatory effects in colon cancer cells. *Human molecular genetics* 2012, 21(10):2157-2165.

[89] Liu PT, Wheelwright M, Teles R, Komisopoulou E, Edfeldt K, Ferguson B, Mehta MD, Vazirnia A, Rea TH, Sarno EN et al: MicroRNA-21 targets the vitamin D-dependent antimicrobial pathway in leprosy. *Nature medicine* 2012, 18(2):267-273.

[90] Karkeni E, Bonnet L, Marcotorchino J, Tourniaire F, Astier J, Ye J, Landrier JF: Vitamin D limits inflammation-linked microRNA expression in adipocytes *in vitro* and *in vivo*: A new mechanism for the regulation of inflammation by vitamin D. *Epigenetics* 2018, 13(2):156-162.

[91] Kasiappan R, Sun Y, Lungchukiet P, Quarni W, Zhang X, Bai W: Vitamin D suppresses leptin stimulation of cancer growth through microRNA. *Cancer research* 2014, 74(21):6194-6204.

[92] Li YC, Chen Y, Liu W, Thadhani R: MicroRNA-mediated mechanism of vitamin D regulation of innate immune response. *The*

Journal of steroid biochemistry and molecular biology 2014, 144 Pt A:81-86.

[93] Mullin GE, Dobs A: Vitamin d and its role in cancer and immunity: a prescription for sunlight. *Nutrition in clinical practice: official publication of the American Society for Parenteral and Enteral Nutrition* 2007, 22(3):305-322.

[94] Bunch BL, Ma Y, Attwood K, Amable L, Luo W, Morrison C, Guru KA, Woloszynska-Read A, Hershberger PA, Trump DL et al: Vitamin D3 enhances the response to cisplatin in bladder cancer through VDR and TAp73 signaling crosstalk. *Cancer medicine* 2019, 8(5):2449-2461.

[95] Fathi N, Ahmadian E, Shahi S, Roshangar L, Khan H, Kouhsoltani M, Maleki Dizaj S, Sharifi S: Role of vitamin D and vitamin D receptor (VDR) in oral cancer. *Biomedicine & pharmacotherapy = Biomedecine & pharmacotherapie* 2019, 109:391-401.

[96] Xie DD, Chen YH, Xu S, Zhang C, Wang DM, Wang H, Chen L, Zhang ZH, Xia MZ, Xu DX et al: Low vitamin D status is associated with inflammation in patients with prostate cancer. *Oncotarget* 2017, 8(13):22076-22085.

[97] Ahmed JH, Makonnen E, Fotoohi A, Yimer G, Seifu D, Assefa M, Tigeneh W, Aseffa A, Howe R, Aklillu E: Vitamin D Status and Association of VDR Genetic Polymorphism to Risk of Breast Cancer in Ethiopia. *Nutrients* 2019, 11(2).

[98] Lopes N, Sousa B, Martins D, Gomes M, Vieira D, Veronese LA, Milanezi F, Paredes J, Costa JL, Schmitt F: Alterations in Vitamin D signalling and metabolic pathways in breast cancer progression: a study of VDR, CYP27B1 and CYP24A1 expression in benign and malignant breast lesions. *BMC cancer* 2010, 10:483.

[99] Mousa A, Naderpoor N, Teede H, Scragg R, de Courten B: Vitamin D supplementation for improvement of chronic low-grade inflammation in patients with type 2 diabetes: a systematic review and meta-analysis of randomized controlled trials. *Nutrition reviews* 2018, 76(5):380-394.

[100] Rodrigues KF, Pietrani NT, Bosco AA, de Sousa MCR, Silva IFO, Silveira JN, Gomes KB: Lower Vitamin D Levels, but Not VDR Polymorphisms, Influence Type 2 Diabetes Mellitus in Brazilian Population Independently of Obesity. *Medicina* 2019, 55(5).

[101] Chagas CE, Borges MC, Martini LA, Rogero MM: Focus on vitamin D, inflammation and type 2 diabetes. *Nutrients* 2012, 4(1):52-67.

[102] Bednarek-Skublewska A, Smolen A, Jaroszynski A, Zaluska W, Ksiazek A: Effects of vitamin D3 on selected biochemical parameters of nutritional status, inflammation, and cardiovascular disease in patients undergoing long-term hemodialysis. *Polskie Archiwum Medycyny Wewnetrznej* 2010, 120(5):167-174.

[103] Pludowski P, Holick MF, Pilz S, Wagner CL, Hollis BW, Grant WB, Shoenfeld Y, Lerchbaum E, Llewellyn DJ, Kienreich K et al: Vitamin D effects on musculoskeletal health, immunity, autoimmunity, cardiovascular disease, cancer, fertility, pregnancy, dementia and mortality-a review of recent evidence. *Autoimmunity reviews* 2013, 12(10):976-989.

[104] Erbas O, Solmaz V, Aksoy D, Yavasoglu A, Sagcan M, Taskiran D: Cholecalciferol (vitamin D 3) improves cognitive dysfunction and reduces inflammation in a rat fatty liver model of metabolic syndrome. *Life sciences* 2014, 103(2):68-72.

[105] Ning C, Liu L, Lv G, Yang Y, Zhang Y, Yu R, Wang Y, Zhu J: Lipid metabolism and inflammation modulated by Vitamin D in liver of diabetic rats. *Lipids in health and disease* 2015, 14:31.

[106] Jahn D, Dorbath D, Schilling AK, Gildein L, Meier C, Vuille-Dit-Bille RN, Schmitt J, Kraus D, Fleet JC, Hermanns HM et al: Intestinal vitamin D receptor modulates lipid metabolism, adipose tissue inflammation and liver steatosis in obese mice. *Biochimica et biophysica acta Molecular basis of disease* 2019, 1865(6):1567-1578.

[107] Hileman CO, Tangpricha V, Sattar A, McComsey GA: Baseline Vitamin D Deficiency Decreases the Effectiveness of Statins in HIV-Infected Adults on Antiretroviral Therapy. *Journal of acquired immune deficiency syndromes* 2017, 74(5):539-547.

[108] Allavena C, Delpierre C, Cuzin L, Rey D, Viget N, Bernard J, Guillot P, Duvivier C, Billaud E, Raffi F: High frequency of vitamin D deficiency in HIV-infected patients: effects of HIV-related factors and antiretroviral drugs. *The Journal of antimicrobial chemotherapy* 2012, 67(9):2222-2230.

[109] Rodriguez M, Daniels B, Gunawardene S, Robbins GK: High frequency of vitamin D deficiency in ambulatory HIV-Positive patients. *AIDS research and human retroviruses* 2009, 25(1):9-14.

[110] Kwan CK, Eckhardt B, Baghdadi J, Aberg JA: Hyperparathyroidism and complications associated with vitamin D deficiency in HIV-infected adults in New York City, New York. *AIDS research and human retroviruses* 2012, 28(9):1025-1032.

[111] Gauzzi MC, Purificato C, Donato K, Jin Y, Wang L, Daniel KC, Maghazachi AA, Belardelli F, Adorini L, Gessani S: Suppressive effect of 1alpha,25-dihydroxyvitamin D3 on type I IFN-mediated monocyte differentiation into dendritic cells: impairment of functional activities and chemotaxis. *Journal of immunology* 2005, 174(1):270-276.

[112] Malim MH: APOBEC proteins and intrinsic resistance to HIV-1 infection. *Philosophical transactions of the Royal Society of London Series B, Biological sciences* 2009, 364(1517):675-687.

[113] Chutiwitoonchai N, Hiyoshi M, Hiyoshi-Yoshidomi Y, Hashimoto M, Tokunaga K, Suzu S: Characteristics of IFITM, the newly identified IFN-inducible anti-HIV-1 family proteins. *Microbes and infection* 2013, 15(4):280-290.

[114] Guzman-Fulgencio M, Garcia-Alvarez M, Berenguer J, Jimenez-Sousa MA, Cosin J, Pineda-Tenor D, Carrero A, Aldamiz T, Alvarez E, Lopez JC et al: Vitamin D deficiency is associated with severity of liver disease in HIV/HCV coinfected patients. *The Journal of infection* 2014, 68(2):176-184.

[115] El-Maouche D, Mehta SH, Sutcliffe CG, Higgins Y, Torbenson MS, Moore RD, Thomas DL, Sulkowski MS, Brown TT: Vitamin D deficiency and its relation to bone mineral density and liver fibrosis in HIV-HCV coinfection. *Antiviral therapy* 2013, 18(2):237-242.

[116] Ye WZ, Reis AF, Velho G: Identification of a novel Tru9 I polymorphism in the human vitamin D receptor gene. *Journal of human genetics* 2000, 45(1):56-57.

[117] Morrison NA, Yeoman R, Kelly PJ, Eisman JA: Contribution of trans-acting factor alleles to normal physiological variability: vitamin D receptor gene polymorphism and circulating osteocalcin. *Proceedings of the National Academy of Sciences of the United States of America* 1992, 89(15):6665-6669.

[118] Morrison NA, Qi JC, Tokita A, Kelly PJ, Crofts L, Nguyen TV, Sambrook PN, Eisman JA: Prediction of bone density from vitamin D receptor alleles. *Nature* 1994, 367(6460):284-287.

[119] Faraco JH, Morrison NA, Baker A, Shine J, Frossard PM: ApaI dimorphism at the human vitamin D receptor gene locus. *Nucleic acids research* 1989, 17(5):2150.

[120] Correa P, Rastad J, Schwarz P, Westin G, Kindmark A, Lundgren E, Akerstrom G, Carling T: The vitamin D receptor (VDR) start codon polymorphism in primary hyperparathyroidism and parathyroid VDR messenger ribonucleic acid levels. *The Journal of clinical endocrinology and metabolism* 1999, 84(5):1690-1694.

[121] Thakkinstian A, D'Este C, Attia J: Haplotype analysis of VDR gene polymorphisms: a meta-analysis. Osteoporosis international: a journal established as result of cooperation between the European Foundation for Osteoporosis and the National Osteoporosis Foundation of the USA 2004, 15(9):729-734.

[122] Slattery ML: Vitamin D receptor gene (VDR) associations with cancer. *Nutrition reviews* 2007, 65(8 Pt 2):S102-104.

[123] Denzer N, Vogt T, Reichrath J: Vitamin D receptor (VDR) polymorphisms and skin cancer: A systematic review. *Dermato-endocrinology* 2011, 3(3):205-210.

[124] Grant DJ, Hoyo C, Akushevich L, Iversen ES, Whitaker R, Marks J, Berchuck A, Schildkraut JM: Vitamin D receptor (VDR) polymorphisms and risk of ovarian cancer in Caucasian and African American women. *Gynecologic oncology* 2013, 129(1):173-178.

[125] Mikhak B, Hunter DJ, Spiegelman D, Platz EA, Hollis BW, Giovannucci E: Vitamin D receptor (VDR) gene polymorphisms and haplotypes, interactions with plasma 25-hydroxyvitamin D and 1,25-dihydroxyvitamin D, and prostate cancer risk. *The Prostate* 2007, 67(9):911-923.

[126] Friedrich M, Meyberg R, Axt-Fliedner R, Villena-Heinsen C, Tilgen W, Schmidt W, Reichrath J: Vitamin D receptor (VDR) expression is not a prognostic factor in cervical cancer. *Anticancer research 2002, 22(1A):299-304.*

[127] Slatter ML, Yakumo K, Hoffman M, Neuhausen S: Variants of the VDR gene and risk of colon cancer (United States). *Cancer causes & control:* CCC 2001, 12(4):359-364.

[128] Singh T, Adams BD: The regulatory role of miRNAs on VDR in breast cancer. *Transcription* 2017, 8(4):232-241.

[129] Moran-Auth Y, Penna-Martinez M, Badenhoop K: VDR FokI polymorphism is associated with a reduced T-helper cell population under vitamin D stimulation in type 1 diabetes patients. *The Journal of steroid biochemistry and molecular biology* 2015, 148:184-186.

[130] Aslani S, Hossein-Nezhad A, Mirzaei K, Maghbooli Z, Afshar AN, Karimi F: VDR FokI polymorphism and its potential role in the pathogenesis of gestational diabetes mellitus and its complications. *Gynecological endocrinology: the official journal of the International Society of Gynecological Endocrinology* 2011, 27 (12):1055-1060.

[131] De Azevedo Silva J, Guimaraes RL, Brandao LA, Araujo J, Segat L, Crovella S, Sandrin-Garcia P: Vitamin D receptor (VDR) gene polymorphisms and age onset in type 1 diabetes mellitus. *Autoimmunity* 2013, 46(6):382-387.

[132] Singh I, Lavania M, Pathak VK, Ahuja M, Turankar RP, Singh V, Sengupta U: VDR polymorphism, gene expression and vitamin D levels in leprosy patients from North Indian population. *PLoS neglected tropical diseases* 2018, 12(11):e0006823.

[133] Mandal D, Reja AH, Biswas N, Bhattacharyya P, Patra PK, Bhattacharya B: Vitamin D receptor expression levels determine the

severity and complexity of disease progression among leprosy reaction patients. *New microbes and new infections* 2015, 6:35-39.

[134] Rusyati LM KI, Sudarsa P: Increased risk of multibacillary leprosy among petient with low plasma vitamin D level. *Journal of global pharma technology* 2018, 10(5):29-34.

[135] Rahman S, Rehn A, Rahman J, Andersson J, Svensson M, Brighenti S: Pulmonary tuberculosis patients with a vitamin D deficiency demonstrate low local expression of the antimicrobial peptide LL-37 but enhanced FoxP3+ regulatory T cells and IgG-secreting cells. *Clinical immunology* 2015, 156(2):85-97.

[136] Yang HF, Zhang ZH, Chang ZQ, Tang KL, Lin DZ, Xu JZ: Vitamin D deficiency affects the immunity against Mycobacterium tuberculosis infection in mice. *Clinical and experimental medicine* 2013, 13(4):265-270.

[137] Junaid K, Rehman A, Jolliffe DA, Saeed T, Wood K, Martineau AR: Vitamin D deficiency associates with susceptibility to tuberculosis in Pakistan, but polymorphisms in VDR, DBP and CYP2R1 do not. *BMC pulmonary medicine* 2016, 16(1):73.

[138] Sinha S, Gupta K, Mandal D, Das BK, Pandey RM: Serum and Bronchoalveolar Lavage Fluid 25(OH)Vitamin D3 Levels in HIV-1 and Tuberculosis: A Cross-Sectional Study from a Tertiary Care Center in North India. *Current HIV research* 2018, 16(2):167-173.

[139] Zhan Y, Jiang L: Status of vitamin D, antimicrobial peptide cathelicidin and T helper-associated cytokines in patients with diabetes mellitus and pulmonary tuberculosis. *Experimental and therapeutic medicine* 2015, 9(1):11-16.

[140] Anandaiah A, Sinha S, Bole M, Sharma SK, Kumar N, Luthra K, Li X, Zhou X, Nelson B, Han X et al: Vitamin D rescues impaired Mycobacterium tuberculosis-mediated tumor necrosis factor release in macrophages of HIV-seropositive individuals through an enhanced Toll-like receptor signaling pathway in vitro. *Infection and immunity* 2013, 81(1):2-10.

[141] Battersby AJ, Kampmann B, Burl S: Vitamin D in early childhood and the effect on immunity to Mycobacterium tuberculosis. *Clinical & developmental immunology* 2012, 2012:430972.

[142] Salamon H, Bruiners N, Lakehal K, Shi L, Ravi J, Yamaguchi KD, Pine R, Gennaro ML: Cutting edge: Vitamin D regulates lipid metabolism in Mycobacterium tuberculosis infection. *Journal of immunology* 2014, 193(1):30-34.

[143] Rusyati LM AM, Wiraguna AA, Puspawati NMD and Sudarsa P Correlation of Serum Vitamin D Receptor Level with Bacterial Index in Multibacillary Leprosy Patients at Sanglah General Hospital, Bali-Indonesia. *Biomedical and pharmacology journal* 2019.

[144] Roy S, Frodsham A, Saha B, Hazra SK, Mascie-Taylor CG, Hill AV: Association of vitamin D receptor genotype with leprosy type. *The Journal of infectious diseases* 1999, 179(1):187-191.

[145] Daniel C, Schlauch T, Zugel U, Steinmeyer A, Radeke HH, Steinhilber D, Stein J: 22-ene-25-oxa-vitamin D: a new vitamin D analogue with profound immunosuppressive capacities. *European journal of clinical investigation* 2005, 35(5):343-349.

[146] Zugel U, Steinmeyer A, May E, Lehmann M, Asadullah K: Immunomodulation by a novel, dissociated Vitamin D analogue. *Experimental dermatology* 2009, 18(7):619-627.

[147] Upton RA, Knutson JC, Bishop CW, LeVan LW: Pharmacokinetics of doxercalciferol, a new vitamin D analogue that lowers parathyroid hormone. *Nephrology, dialysis, transplantation: official publication of the European Dialysis and Transplant Association - European Renal Association* 2003, 18(4):750-758.

[148] Kakuda S, Okada K, Eguchi H, Takenouchi K, Hakamata W, Kurihara M, Takimoto-Kamimura M: Structure of the ligand-binding domain of rat VDR in complex with the nonsecosteroidal vitamin D3 analogue YR301. *Acta crystallographica Section F, Structural biology and crystallization communications* 2008, 64(Pt 11):970-973.

BIOGRAPHICAL SKETCH

Dibyakanti Mandal

Affiliation: Faculty of life Sciences, Department of Biochemistry, PDM University, Haryana, India

Education:

- PhD (2003) in biochemistry, Calcutta University, Kolkata, India
- MSc (1995) in biochemistry, Calcutta University
- BSc (1993) in Chemistry (Honors), Calcutta University

Professional Appointments:

- Assistant professor, Biochemistry (2019- Till date): PDM University, Haryana, India
- Senior program officer (Oct 2017- Nov 2018): INCLEN Trust, New Delhi, India. Led and coordinated INSPIRE study (pneumococcal conjugate vaccine (PCV) impact in India).
- Senior program officer (July 2016-Sept 2017): Translational Health Sciences and Technology Institute (THSTI), Faridabad, India. Worked on maternal influenza and RSV immunization in India (Gap analysis, preparation of roadmap, develop project proposal).
- Scientist B (September 2015-June 2016): All India Institute of Medical Sciences (AIIMS), New Delhi. Worked on HIV pathogenesis.
- Visiting associate professor (Feb 2014-August 2015): Institute of Genetic Engineering, Kolkata, India. Teaching/research at graduate and postgraduate levels.
- Research Scientist (April 2011-May 2013): University of Iowa. IA. Worked on a) ZFN and TALEN based gene therapy against cystic fibrosis. b) Understanding the pathogenesis of influenza and RSV.

- Research Associate (November 2006-April 2011): University of Iowa, IA, USA: Worked on HIV-1 RNA splicing and regulation of gene expression.
- Post-doctoral fellow (July 2002 – November 2006): Albert Einstein College of Medicine. NY, USA: Worked on molecular determinants of HIV-1 reverse transcriptase functions with a view to further drug development against HIV.
- Visiting fellow (UNECO-IUMS-MIRCENS-SGM Fellowship) (Feb 2002-Apr 2002): Worked on immune response against HIV-1 subtype C envelope gene of Indian isolates. New York University School of Medicine, NY, USA.

Honors:

- 1996: Junior research fellowship awarded by Department of Biotechnology, Govt. of India.
- 2001: Senior research fellowship awarded by Council of Scientific and Industrial research (CSIR), India.
- 2001: UNESCO-IUMS-MIRSENS-SGM international fellowship..
- 2008: Levitt center pilot grant obtained from University of Iowa, Project title: 'Effects of unspliced RNA levels on HIV-1 Gag assembly'.

Publications (last 3 years):

A. Peer-reviewed publications:

1) Sinha S, Agarwal A, Gupta K, Mandal D, Jain M, Detels R, Nandy K, DeVos MA, Sharma SK, Manoharan N, Julka PK, Rath GK· Ambinder RF, Mitsuyasu RT. 2018. Prevalence of HIV in patients with malignancy and of malignancy in HIV patients in a tertiary care center from North India. *Curr HIV Res.* 2018 Oct 18.
2) Sinha S, Gupta K, Nawaid Khan, Mandal D, et al. 2018. Higher frequency of HIV-1 drug resistance and increased NRTI mutations

among the HIV-1 positive ART naive individuals co-infected with Mycobacterium Tuberculosis compared to only HIV infection in India. *Infectious Disease: Research and Treatment.*

3) Sinha S, Gupta K, Mandal D, Das BK, Pandey RM. 2018. Serum and Bronchoalveolar Lavage Fluid 25(OH) Vitamin D3 Levels in HIV-1 and Tuberculosis: A Cross-Sectional Study from a Tertiary Care Center in North India. *Curr HIV Res.* 27.

B. Conference abstracts:

1) Mandal D and DJ Chattopadhaya. Interferon induced transmembrane protein (IFITM) restricts Chandipura and Respiratory Syncytial Virus. 5th Molecular Virology Meeting. Feb 11-12, 2017. THSTI, Faridabad.

2) Sanjeev Sinha, Dibyakanti Mandal, Pooja Kasana Assessment of the Role of Bronchoalveolar Lavage Fluid (BALF) and Serum Vitamin D Levels in AIDS Disease Progression and Opportunistic Infections Amongst HIV and Tuberculosis Co-Infected Individuals. *American Journal of Respiratory and Critical Care Medicine* 2016;193:A5522.

INDEX

C

D

E

F

G

H

I

K

L

M

N

O

P

R

S

T

U

V

W

Related Nova Publications

SALMONELLA ENTERICA: MOLECULAR CHARACTERIZATION, ROLE IN INFECTIOUS DISEASES AND EMERGING RESEARCH

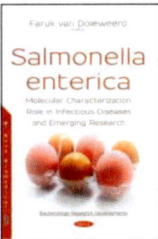

EDITOR: Faruk van Doleweerd

SERIES: Bacteriology Research Developments

BOOK DESCRIPTION: The bacterium Salmonella enterica is a serious bacterial pathogen and causative agent of salmonellosis infections on a worldwide scale.

SOFTCOVER ISBN: 978-1-53613-084-3
RETAIL PRICE: $82

CELLULAR INTERACTIONS OF PROBIOTIC BACTERIA WITH INTESTINAL AND IMMUNE CELLS

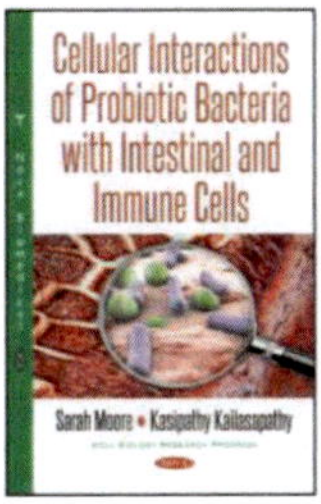

AUTHORS: Sarah Moore and Kasipathy Kailasapathy

SERIES: Bacteriology Research Developments

BOOK DESCRIPTION: This book contains novel research and laboratory techniques to study the immune cell molecular behaviour and responses to soluble factors produced by probiotic bacteria and intestinal/probiotic co-cultures that will contribute to advanced scientific knowledge and the commercial development of probiotics.

HARDCOVER ISBN: 978-1-53612-172-8
RETAIL PRICE: $160

To see a complete list of Nova publications, please visit our website at www.novapublishers.com

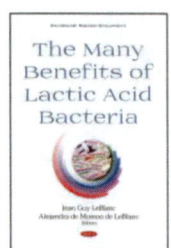

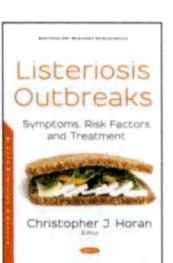